'This is an important book. John Ashton shows how and why the catastrophic actions of Boris Johnson's government failed its people and led to many thousands of unnecessary deaths. If we are to avoid similar disasters, read this scorching indictment of those in power.'
KEN LOACH

'In 1847 the much celebrated and revered Doctor William Henry Duncan was appointed as Liverpool's first Medical Officer of Health. Like Dr Duncan, and motivated by a passion for the common good, John Ashton sees the world through the lens of public health. From the outset of the Coronavirus pandemic he has offered trenchant and coherent arguments about how the Government and public-health authorities needed to respond. His insightful book provides a valuable compass and road map as we continue to navigate our way through this pandemic. He also offers sound advice on how to be better prepared for fresh waves of Covid and other potential threats to public health. As Dr Duncan might have said—just what the doctor ordered.'
LORD ALTON

'John Ashton has been the voice of Cassandra throughout the pandemic. He has earned the right to be the first to tell the whole story, showing that we had both experience and knowledge, but failed to use it. But in the face of the arrogance of centralisation, Ashton gives us hope that local communities and expertise are equipped to bring the 2020 pandemic to its conclusion.'
CRISPIN PAILING

BLINDED BY CORONA

This first edition published in the UK in 2020 by Gibson Square.

ISBN: 9781783341955
email: rights@gibsonsquare.com
website: www.gibsonsquare.com

Cover image: Peter Dredge.

Papers used by Gibson Square are natural, recyclable products made from wood grown in sustainable forests; inks used are vegetable based. Manufacturing conforms to ISO 14001, and is accredited to FSC and PEFC chain of custody schemes. Colour-printing is through a certified CarbonNeutral® company that offsets its CO2 emissions.

BLINDED

BY

CORONA

JOHN ASHTON
with Maggi Morris

GIBSON SQUARE

'Man has lost the capacity to foresee and to forestall,
he will end by destroying the world.'
Albert Schweitzer

'You are the hollow man
You are the stuffed man
Leaning together
Headpiece filled with straw. Alas!'
With apologies to T S Eliot.

'We are less aware that it breeds folly; that the power to command frequently
causes failure to think; that the responsibility of power often fades as its
exercise augments. The overall responsibility of power is to govern as
reasonably as possible in the interest of the state and its citizens. A duty in
that process is to keep well-informed, to heed information, to keep mind and
judgement open and to resist the insidious spell of wooden-headedness. If the
mind is open enough to perceive that a given policy is harming rather than
serving self-interest, and self-confident enough to acknowledge it, and wise
enough to reverse it, that is the summit in the art of government.'
Barbara Tuchman
The March of Folly: From Troy to Vietnam

CONTENTS

In public health, even if you don't have direct control over a threat to the population's health, you have to assure yourself it is being dealt with. If you find that isn't the case then your next job is to bring together those who do have control and coordinate an effective response.

This book is dedicated to the memory of William Henry Duncan, Medical Officer of Health for Liverpool 1847-63 and to his successors around the world who speak truth to power to protect the health of the people. That is the highest law.

Blinded by Corona

The year 2020 will go down in world history as the 'Year of the COVID-19 Pandemic', taking its place in the annals of public health, alongside the Black Death of the fourteenth century, the Great Plague of London of 1665, the so-called 'Spanish 'flu' of 1919 and other major epidemics that have swept the world both before and since with enormous loss of life, together with tumultuous economic and political ramifications.

What is different about COVID is that it had been long anticipated and that despite a century of an ascendant medical science and a rhetoric of preparedness, many countries were caught out. Not least among them was the UK.

To understand the root causes of this catastrophic failure it is necessary to address seventy years of neglect of the public-health system since the Second World War and to recognise that the very success of scientific medicine over that time brought with it the seeds of this major public-health disaster. It is also important to make the connection between biological phenomena like the pandemic and the way we live on the planet with global economies, rapid urbanisation and their impacts on biological systems and sustainability. We inhabit the earth on sufferance with no inalienable right to survive more than other animal species that have come and gone. The story of COVID-19 is a story of hubris, the hubris of humans as a species, together with the hubris of political and scientific leaders who lacked the humility to ask themselves the difficult questions early enough and to be open and transparent with the public.

The British government, under the recently elected Prime Minister Boris Johnson, was caught flat-footed and stands accused of doing too little, too late. When it comes to the specific COVID-19 failings of the Johnson cabinet and its scientific advisers in the United Kingdom we might reflect, with Tolstoy, that successful countries are all alike whilst every unsuccessful country is unsuccessful in its own way and that tens of thousands of British people have almost certainly died wantonly.

It is the dream of scientists to defeat the pathogens and other agents that can wreak havoc in human populations. With each victory the hope is that a definitive blow has been dealt in the fight to ward of illness. In the scientific age the hospital has come to replace the cathedral as the focus of hope for eternal life.

This dream is especially grandiose when it comes to ever evolving infectious diseases that can be found in the reservoir of other species that we come into contact with as we exploit the natural environment for our own comfort and convenience. After we have managed to control and suppress an epidemic, perhaps with the aid of a vaccine and modern medicines, there is a feeling of congratulation and invincibility.

Too often scientists and politicians seem to forget that in a world population of 8 billion sharing habitats and environments with multiple other species, from other mammals to the humblest but most versatile of simple life forms such as RNA viruses, respect for nature is a prerequisite for survival. René Dubos, the American microbiologist and author of *Mirage of Health*, who coined the phrase 'Think globally, act locally', reminded us that 'at some unpredictable time, and in some unforeseeable manner, nature will strike back'.

The known unknown is that there will be another epidemic, and later another, and another. Just what isn't known is the why, how, and when before it is too late. There will be no sabre-rattling beforehand and how well a population can mitigate an epidemic will depend on its preparedness, resilience and public mobilisation acting in concert with the evidence and the science. The advantage that nature will always have over mankind is the element of surprise and the arrogance of leaders who think they have all the answers.

I have spent over forty years in a public-health career encompassing academia as well as hands-on public-health practice at all levels; from the neighbourhood to the global with the World Health Organization, I have dealt with a wide range of major public-health emergencies and knew that one day the world would face a crisis on the scale of the Influenza pandemic of 1918-19. What none of us knew was whether it would be in our lifetime.

When the first news broke of the unfolding epidemic in China it seemed possible that this might be the big one. It felt necessary to sound the alarm in the interview I gave to Sky News on February 1, outside Arrowe Park Hospital on the Wirral, Merseyside, as the first returnees from Wuhan went into quarantine there, and the first cases were reported in York.

My comments then were, 'What we are seeing now are the first couple of cases in York, there are likely to be more. With these situations it's like the millennial bug when we took a lot of precautions coming up to 2000 to stop computers crashing. When it didn't happen people said "what a waste of money". You have to be prepared. You have to put the effort in and if it doesn't happen — great! People should be concerned in order to take action.'

My official involvement with the global response was not in the UK but started in the second week of February when I was contacted by the Crown Prince of Bahrain to give advice on the country's response to the Corona threat. He had watched the Sky News broadcast on February 1 and wished to assure himself that his country was prepared and that the country's response that was being put in place would be robust.

Crown Prince Salman, who was also the First Deputy Prime Minister and deputy commander of the Bahrain army, had been alert to the threat of the new virus from mid-January. On February 3 he had set up a Task Force in a dedicated War Room with an extensive multidisciplinary team, led clinically by Lt-Colonel Dr Manaf Al-Quatani.

Prince Salman asked me to examine the Task Force's arrangements forensically and to identify any weak points in the chain of defence against the virus and its threat to the people of Bahrain. Over two visits in February and March, and subsequently via Skype calls as Britain was locked down, I became embedded within the Task Force and had the immense satisfaction of being able to make recommendations that were in the most part immediately acted on. The Crown Prince's team brought home an impressive victory against the pandemic, being praised by the Director General of the World Health Organization for its response. It ranks among the best in the world in creating an effective blueprint.

Meanwhile I was taken aback to see what was happening in the UK in comparison to Bahrain. No country could have been fully ready for what was coming in January 2020, especially with a novel virus as contagious and potentially lethal as COVID-19. Also, the proud tradition of public health in the UK, but especially in England, had suffered body blows with ten years of austerity and chaotic structural reforms in 2013. The country went into the crisis with a dysfunctional scientific advisory system and an over-centralised public-health agency, Public Health England (PHE). Nevertheless, at the heart of it was a highly skilled public-health and NHS workforce with some outstanding local leadership standing ready to respond as if in the Battle of Stalingrad from street to street, house to house, workplace to workplace.

What followed was shocking. Unlike what happened in Bahrain, Britain's NHS and public-health teams were failed by the lack of prompt and effective leadership at the top, political, professional and organisational. There is still zero interest in a coherent plan to fight the pandemic efficiently and effectively. To this day, all we get is an initiative that is good for a column headline: here today, gone tomorrow.

What the NHS and the Public Health Service needed and need is attentive, competent direction. Instead Boris Johnson—flanked by Dominic Cummings, Dominic Raab and Matt Hancock—was in charge. By so-called 'Independence Day' on July 4 an estimated 65,000 people had perished in the UK from COVID-19, about half of them in the nation's care homes. A majority of these deaths could have been avoided. In addition, much of the harm to the economy, education, medical care for those with illnesses, social care for the aged and vulnerable, and the nation's health in general, that came from the ensuing lockdown might have been averted. Instead, England suffered unnecessarily on these fronts and others that may yet open up.

Six months into the pandemic, Johnson's cabinet had the worst results of all G20 countries, if not the world—apart from Belgium. The country that invented epidemiology was still struggling with what to do about COVID—apart from chancellor Rishi Sunak borrowing up to half a trillion pounds according to Office of National Statistics estimates in order to offer tax breaks, fund businesses' payrolls and other indirect pandemic monies. It was announced on 17 August that the name Public Health England would disappear to be replaced with a plaque called National Institute for Health Protection. Writing cheques, changing words, and musical chairs for two of London's civil-servants, however, did not amount to a wrench against the pandemic's attack on Britain's health and wealth.

The future remains uncertain. We know much more than at the beginning of the pandemic. But with a novel virus such as COVID-19 many aspects remain a mystery. Whether it will just fade away as did its near relative and the cause of SARS (Severe, Acute Respiratory Syndrome) in 2003, or return in further waves, either more or less severe, we have yet to find out. In July there was a resurgence of the pandemic looking likely in many countries and the failure to squash it to zero levels of infection in England and Wales. There were dozens of local outbreaks.

It is to chronicle what we could have done and what we did do, the tragedy of errors, that prompted this book. Specifically, there are the factors that created in Britain the greatest systemic public-health failures of all time at the beginning of the crisis. Separately, there is the absentee leadership once the crisis got going. A reasonably competent leadership would have dealt with legacy issues head on rather than with their head in the clouds. The public inquiry that has been announced will need to examine both these aspects on their own.

During the COVID pandemic many people have lost and many more will regretfully yet lose loved ones. This book is also written to give them an insight into the question whether the Johnson cabinet rose to the occasion, or let their relatives down with tragic consequences.

1

Plagues in History

The idea of epidemics as 'plagues' has a provenance dating back to the book of Exodus in the Old Testament of the Bible. There the term was used generically to apply to catastrophic events, including a population being overwhelmed by frogs, lice, boils and locusts among the ten disasters inflicted on Egypt by the God of Israel to force the Pharaoh into allowing the Israelites to escape from slavery.

It was not until the sixth century, with the first recorded pandemic of infectious disease, that the term acquired a connotation that is understandable in terms of modern biological knowledge. That Justinian plague from 541-549 AD, caused by the bacterium Yersinia Pestis was carried by rat fleas and spread on board ships throughout the Mediterranean and Near East. With the centre of the epidemic in Constantinople, the disease affected the Roman Emperor, Justinian, who recovered from it, but it killed an estimated fifth of the capital's population. However, probably the two best known outbreaks of the plague in the western world are the Black Death of the fourteenth century and the Great Plague of London of 1665-66, immortalised in Daniel Defoe's *Journal of the Plague Year* published in 1722.

The Black Death, or Bubonic Plague, also carried by infected fleas, is claimed to have been the most fatal pandemic in human history. Deaths are estimated at between 75-200 million worldwide including over one third of the European population, having arrived in Europe via the trade routes from Asia. The pattern of the clinical infection was unremitting, causing inflamed lymph glands or 'buboes' especially in the groin, swollen tongues, spitting headaches, severe vomiting and blackening of the skin, generally leading to an agonising death.

200 years later, when the Great Plague of London decimated the population, the epidemic spread from overcrowded parish to overcrowded parish in the rapidly growing city, with escalating death rates, especially among the poor. The wealthy fled to their country properties where they could, taking the infection with them to smaller towns and rural areas. The most notorious rural outbreak was in the village of Eyam, in Derbyshire, where 80% of the villagers died having stayed put and self- quarantined to avoid spreading the plague to other settlements.

In Defoe's retrospective account there was speculation among Londoners that the causes of the plague went beyond the over-crowding of the slums to more mystical, religious and magical explanations as foretold by the appearance of comets and stars. Other aspects of Defoe's observations that have resonance with recent experience with COVID-19 include efforts to certify people as free from disease to allow them to travel; measures put in place to achieve social distancing by pedestrians walking down the centre of highways to avoid affected households; the challenges of mass burial, and arguments about the validity of death statistics. Defoe noted that the numbers of ordinary burials in which plague was not mentioned as a cause of death, increased substantially during the period of the epidemic in those parishes most affected, drawing attention in effect to the greater validity of measuring all-cause mortality in assessing its impact.

However in terms of plague literature it is Albert Camus' novel *The Plague* that provides the most enigmatic account. Set in Oran, a coastal town in Algeria, where the writer had lived, the novel explores many themes of an epidemic in a closed community in lockdown which have become familiar during the COVID emergency. These include vacillation over calling the epidemic, conflicts over quarantine and the lockdown itself, the vulnerability of the poor and disadvantaged, the pain of separation, complacency and hubris, the role of religious assembly in disease transmission, censorship of the press and news management, arguments over the science, the handling of mass funerals and rows about calling an end to the epidemic.

Although it is these well-known and devastating, large scale epidemics that have captured popular imagination, other infectious diseases have periodically demanded concerted action by governments and later by international agencies. Historically outbreaks have often been associated with population movements and mixing relating to trade, colonial exploitation, war, and travel for leisure, especially when travellers have introduced previously unexposed populations to new infectious agents.

Whilst it is true to say that in most wars disease accounts for more deaths than the actual fighting, it is especially the case that venereal infection is strongly associated with military mobilisation. Syphilis seems to have been brought back to Europe by Columbus's 1492 expedition to the New World leading to an outbreak in the French army during the battle of Naples of 1495 and was second only to the Spanish 'flu as a cause of sickness absence among American troops in World War I. Such were the levels of venereal infection among British troops returning from the trenches in 1919 that a network of special clinics was established by local authorities to treat the long term complications.

In 1778 measles was believed to be introduced into the Pacific islands by Captain Cook's voyages and has been blamed for the crash of Tahiti's population from 135,000 in 1820 to around

60,000 a hundred years later. However it was the regular pandemics of cholera that emanated from Asia and spread by maritime trade to the burgeoning slums of industrialising Western countries that provided the impetus for the development of the Victorian public-health movement, leaving an international legacy of institutional arrangements, not least in the UK which was in the vanguard.

The Great Influenza of 1919, 'The Spanish 'flu'

While accounts such as those by Defoe and Camus provide insights into the social, political and cultural impacts of a pandemic caused by a bacterium, it is the so-called Spanish 'flu of 1918-1920 that provides the first chronicled example of a virus wreaking havoc at a global scale. The most likely origin of what has been called 'The Great Influenza' was in the rural and poverty stricken county of Haskell, in Texas, in 1918.

In his comprehensive description of the lead up to the outbreak and subsequent course of the pandemic as it went global, John Barry recounts how a handful of cases of a most virulent strain of influenza were first brought to the attention of Loring Miner, an unusual rural doctor with a taste for the classics.

A man rather in the tradition of the celebrated Wensleydale general practitioner, Will Pickles, who charted the spread of childhood infections such as measles through his country practice in the Yorkshire Dales in the 1930's, Miner was a medical scientist before such a breed had barely taken root in the US. In January and early February of 1918, he saw a succession of patients who were brought down with violent headaches and body aches, a high fever and a non-productive cough, killing many of them. Dr Miner, who was ahead of his time in having created his own, small laboratory in the practice, explored the blood, urine and sputum of his patients in a desperate effort to identify the causes of the illness, searched the literature, discussed with colleagues, and reported his experience to the US Public Health Service. The latter, according to Barry, offered him neither assistance nor advice. And then the disease seemingly disappeared.

The influenza soon reappeared in a large military camp 300 miles away where thousands of young recruits were being mobilised to join the allied forces in Europe for the final phases of World War I. In a bitterly cold winter and in overcrowded, underheated conditions, where they were huddled together for warmth, these and hundreds of thousands of brother squaddies in many similar camps across the country, had been cooped up waiting for mobilisation.

At the beginning of March, the same clinical picture that Dr Miner had seen in Haskell began to emerge here, and later other camps, and ravaged through the troops. Before long it seems to have travelled with them into the battlefields of France and Belgium and soon impacted on the German troops, if anything with greater ferocity (possibly contributing to their failure to secure victory).

The virus subsequently returned to the US, as it did to all corners of the world, becoming known as the 'Spanish 'flu' only because censorship in the field of war had failed to report its Texan antecedents.

The tendency to blame other countries for epidemic diseases is a well-established one, not least when they carry a social stigma as in the case of venereal infection, syphilis most notoriously having been known as French pox in England and the English Disease in France. The habit of attributing geographical labels with political connotations to epidemics of viral pneumonia would be something that would arouse great emotion with COVID-19. By the time of the last Spanish 'flu victim in December 1920, the pandemic had accounted for between 50 and 100 million lives worldwide. A distinguishing feature of the pandemic was that its victims tended to be much younger than those normally affected by influenza viruses.

Barry's account reminds us that a century ago virology was in its infancy, as indeed was scientific medicine, and that the American medical schools had only recently emerged from domination by quackery and religion with the establishment of Johns Hopkins University in 1876. *The Great Influenza* provides rich insights into the personalities, characters, competitiveness, strengths and weaknesses, foibles and peccadilloes of many of the giants of American medicine of the times as they struggled to throw light on the nature of the new virus. For much of the time they were thrown off track by the unusual clinical presentation of atypical pneumonia that also affected a range of other organs and systems beside the lungs; something that resonates with the experience of COVID-19, perhaps even now raising questions as to the diagnostic accuracy at that time.

The virus involved in the 1919 pandemic has long been held to have belonged to the influenza group of viruses and therefore different from the coronavirus, COVID-19, but in many ways, in addition to its multi-organ clinical presentations it bears an uncanny resemblance. Not only did the 1918-19 pandemic creep up silently on an unprepared world but its social, political and economic impact provided a foretaste of what the world is grappling with in 2020.

Hesitancy and resistance in the face of a growing emergency, a weak public-health system and a political leader, President Woodrow Wilson, preoccupied by his sense of mission towards Europe, albeit a desire to join the war to defeat Germany rather than a battle for Brexit, distracted attention from the enemy virus within the USA that was biding its time, ready to wreak havoc on an unknowing world.

Wilson's single-minded focus on the war effort enabled mass gatherings to take place that undoubtedly seeded the initial epidemic around the country, together with a succession of unmonitored marine sea movements of troops and merchant vessels plying between the ports and army camps of the eastern seaboard.

One day we may know whether among the main SAGE advisers to the UK government there was a public-health historian. It doesn't seem likely.

2

Straws in the Wind

'Problems worthy of attack, prove their worth by hitting back.'
Piet Hein, Danish polymath

It is crucial to understand the evolution of human urbanisation in order to understand modern epidemics in general and COVID-19 in particular. The history of patterns of health and disease in human populations is intimately bound up with it.

The population of England and Wales in 1086 was of the order of 1.25 million, as estimated in the Domesday Book. For the next 600 years there was slow overall growth, interrupted by dramatic decline caused by the Black Death, and by 1695 the population stood at about 5.5 million. Accurate figures are available from the decennial census that has been conducted since 1801 when the population was nearly 9 million. The population doubled in the first half of the nineteenth century and nearly doubled again in the second half to about 35 million. Over one million British military personnel perished during both world wars. After 1901 the population increase slowed with deferment of the birth of first children, dramatic reductions in family size towards one- or two-child families and a significant proportion of women, perhaps as high as 20%, electing to have no children or being childless at the end of the childbearing years.

What drove the quadrupling? The possible explanations for a

change in population size include a positive balance of migration, an increase in the birth-rate or a decline in the death-rate. Historically migration does not appear to have been an important factor until recently, and it is unlikely that the population increase before the middle of the nineteenth century was caused by an increasing birth rate. This was already high and had begun to decline in the latter part of the century; it is more likely that the dramatic increase in population was accounted for by a reduction in death rates, especially among children. Significant immigration of younger workers from Europe and beyond has been the main contributor to increases in the overall population in recent decades.

The overall effect of demographic trends since the World War II, and especially since the 1970's, has been a dramatic change in the age distribution of the population with many fewer children and young people together with a much greater proportion of people living well beyond the biblical three score years and ten, into their 80's, 90's and beyond. These trends have not been distributed equally with corresponding growing gaps opening up in both life expectancy and healthy life expectancy between the most fortunate and the most disadvantaged.

During most of the existence of the human race a large proportion of all children probably died in the first few years of life. The sustained reductions in deaths from the eighteenth century onwards have to a large extent been attributable to reduction in the toll from infectious diseases associated with nutritional and environmental factors. Simply put, healthier nutrition and more hygienic environment shrank the national death-rate from infection for infants. The most important of these have been tuberculosis, chest infections, and the water- and food-borne diarrhoeal diseases.

Paradoxically, it meant that the share of deaths caused by infection grew among the entire population. The predominance of infectious disease as a cause of death probably dates from the rapid urbanisation and creation of urban slums that followed the agricultural and industrial revolutions. In this sense the disturbance of longstanding human habitats with disruption of the relationship between people and their environments, thrown together into overcrowded slums, was critical in creating fertile conditions in which epidemic disease could become established and spread. We see the same in parts of the world that are currently urbanising.

Particularly the underprivileged benefitted from local public-health management. During the nineteenth century, increased food production stemming from changes in agriculture led to significant nutritional benefits and later reduced family size from the widespread adoption of birth control has been a significant factor in improving the prospects of children from poorer households by increasing their share of available resources including food. From the 1840's onwards the systematic public-health responses of local public-health teams based in the town hall and supported by central government, substantially designed out many of the environmental conditions that undermined healthy living. This was achieved through close working relationships with town planners producing a wide range of initiatives such as slum improvement and the building of council housing, the provision of safe water and sanitation, paving of streets and refuse collection, the creation of urban parks, and wash houses.

Today, all of these are all taken for granted and considered preconditions of a robust economy. But it is good to remember at one point or another, they were controversial public-health initiatives that had to overcome government inertia if not staunch resistance of those who thought they knew better or that the status quo was good enough.

What is remarkable to many is the recognition that, with the exception of vaccination against smallpox, it is unlikely that immunisation or medical treatment had a significant impact on mortality from infectious disease before the twentieth century. In particular, and a most important message when we come to consider COVID-19, most of the reduction in mortality from tuberculosis, bronchitis, pneumonia and influenza, whooping cough and food and water-borne diseases had already occurred before effective immunisation or treatment was available.

To those who think a COVID-vaccine will be the silver bullet this recognition may give some pause for thought. It is only since the advances in scientific medicine and pharmacology after World War II that the contributions from these two fields of endeavour have been able to take their meaningful place alongside those from environmental, political, economic and social measures. Even so, the operative words are 'take their meaningful place alongside', not by any stretch of the imagination 'replace'.

Since World War II the remarkable progress in scientific medicine has delivered huge benefits to population health, not least through the development of an extensive range of vaccinations that have all but eliminated many of the childhood infectious diseases that used to kill and maim thousands every year. Measles, mumps, rubella, polio, diphtheria, whooping cough, and some forms of meningitis are among those that were much feared by previous generations of parents and tuberculosis, smallpox, epidemic pneumonia and winter seasonal 'flu have all been significantly reduced in their impact through the application of vaccination in countries with well-developed health systems.

Nevertheless the shadow of the Spanish Influenza Pandemic of 1918-19 has always hung around in the background. There have been regular reminders of the possibility of a future return by lesser pandemics in 1957 and 1968, both believed to have originated in Asia, which caused respectively one million and as many as four million deaths worldwide. These three outbreaks have been attributed to three different antigenic subtypes of the influenza group A virus: H1N1, H2N2, and H3H2, respectively. In addition an epidemic of H1N1 in 1951, originating in Liverpool, accounted for more weekly deaths in the city than had occurred in 1919 and the most deaths in one week since the cholera epidemic of 1849, only exceeded by those from aerial bombardment during the May blitz of the docklands in 1941.

What makes the influenza strains so different compared to the more manageable infectious diseases? One of the challenges that 'flu viruses pose to public health is that these simple life forms are constantly evolving and mutating, such that any immunity that has been acquired from exposure to a previous strain may be useless when a novel variant emerges.

Medical science is just not as nimble as the virus itself. Efforts to anticipate the circulating strains of virus and pre-empt serious outbreaks have come to take the form of influenza vaccines containing the three or four most prevalent strains with the ambition of achieving high population levels of vaccination coverage each year in the winter 'flu season. Despite energetic efforts, coverage levels vary and a significant toll of deaths and complications is a regular feature of the winter period in many countries, affecting usually older, more vulnerable people and those suffering from pre-existing medical conditions. Typically several hundred thousands of people perish globally each year from seasonal influenza, representing a mortality rate of below 0.1% of those affected.

It is worth, therefore, noting that immediately effective low-cost public-health solutions are available apart from not entirely reliable medical wizardry. Simply wearing face masks when symptomatic, or washing hands frequently, are impressively effective hygienic barriers to curb the spread of such diseases through aerosols or touch. A common refrain against public health is that it is impossible to change habits of a lifetime. But one only has to point at Britain's sustained campaign regarding smoking habits to see what is possible if one makes a start.

The belief that the advent of modern medicine together with immunisation and vaccination was leading to the demise of infectious disease was in part behind the post-war rundown of public health in many countries, not least in the UK. The abolition of the local-government post of Medical Officer of Health in 1974 and the move of public health into the National Health Service was followed in 1988 by serious failures of response that led to the deaths of 19 patients from *salmonella* food poisoning at the Stanley Royd psychogeriatric hospital in Wakefield and of 22 patients from *legionella* at Stafford hospital resulting from poor links between the NHS and environmental health in local government. Later in the year a major national epidemic of *salmonella* in poultry eggs became a national scandal that ended the career of junior health minister Edwina Currie and resulted in the slaughter of 4 million hens.

The importance of this period in time and its relevance to COVID in 2020 is in demonstrating the delicate and potentially explosive relationship between political and technical advice on public health matters and whether the science informs the politics or whether the politics shapes the expression of the science.

Putting all eggs in a medical-science basket probably seemed smart as a matter of trimming public expenditure. But it was penny-wise pound foolish and no lessons were drawn from these scandals whose national, economic impact belied their local origins. Although some measures were taken by the Chief Medical Officer of the time, Sir Donald Acheson, to strengthen public health, the under-valuing of public health in Britain continued.

The *salmonella* and *legionella* incidents were but a foretaste of what was to come, not least from a series of novel infections and variants on the old theme of Influenza and other viruses. HIV, with a 100% death rate, was followed a few years later by Bovine Spongiform Encephalitis, BSE or Mad Cow Disease, which led to exposure of the population at large. Caused by an unusual pathogenic organism known as a prion and associated with the recycling of animal meat into the foodstuffs of herbivores, it had appeared in 1986, again with a devastating agricultural impact and serious political ramifications. Hong Kong or Avian 'flu occurred in 1997, caused by the H5N1 virus; Severe Acute Respiratory Syndrome, caused by the SARS-CoV virus, a relative of COVID-19, in 2003; Swine 'flu, caused by subtypes of the influenza A virus, including H1N1, H3N2, and H2N3 in 2009; and in 2014, Ebola, a severe viral haemorrhaging fever with high infectivity and very high mortality, caused by the virus EBV, and emerging from the same area of sub-Saharan Africa as the HIV virus which had gone global in the 1980's with the loss of almost one million people at the most recent count. In 2001 a massive outbreak of foot-and-mouth disease in cattle affected herds across the country. To prevent them entering the human food chain tens of thousands were slaughtered and cremated with devastating impact on farm economies and the mental health of farm workers.

We will return to more detail below, but if ever there was truth in Piet Hein's short poem at the beginning of this chapter it was contained in this succession of left-field viral attacks on Britain's population and the enormous costs they left in their wake.

Britain's shoe-leather public-health response
At its best, the long tradition of public health in Britain can trace its roots back 200 years to the practical application of 'shoe leather epidemiology' in the cholera epidemics of the 1840's and 50's. The pioneering work of the country's first Medical Officer of Health, William Henry Duncan, in Liverpool is a reference point for all public-health students. He tackled the 1849 cholera epidemic in the city together with his colleagues, sanitary engineer Thomas Fresh and borough engineer James Newlands. There is also the much celebrated work of John Snow in London, whose detective work during the 1854 epidemic led to the handle being taken off

a street-water pump, ending the outbreak in Broad Street. The late Geoffrey Rose, clinical epidemiologist at the London School of Hygiene and Tropical Medicine, summed up their ethos succinctly. To be effective in public health it is necessary to have 'a clean mind and dirty hands'. It is a tradition that has been the root of all practise of public health down the generations in Britain.

Health-emergency planners categorise emergencies into one of three types: the Slow Burn, the Rising Tide, or the Big Bang. That is not to say that there is one characteristic they all share. If the planners are permitted to do their job well, and prevent a lethal catastrophe, there will be a loud chorus of nay-sayers clamouring about the measures that were taken, 'What was all that about?' As happened with the Millennium Bug, the absence of mayhem is taken as proof after the fact that there was no emergency. This reaction is practically a given in public health. It is part of human nature and there is no easy answer to it. A false positive—an emergency response to virus that turns out not to have the virulence to cause a global pandemic—will dial down the public-health approach to the next emergency as we will see with Ebola.

Whilst each major incident is unique in its own way, and has its own 'battle rhythm', triage of the emergency can usually be established within a very short space of time after the first occurrence. The combination of epidemiological description together with shoe-leather epidemiology and social science in the form of applied anthropology proved to be crucial in unravelling the mystery of HIV/AIDS, an extraordinarily lethal virus, when it first came to attention around 1980 among gay men in North America.

In the case of HIV/AIDS the pandemic initially had the characteristics of a 'Slow Burn'. Through most of the developed world there was initially little interest in a novel disease that seemed to only affect a stigmatised minority of gay men. It was of little interest to mainstream clinicians and researchers, the pharmaceutical industry, politicians, the mass media or the general public. It was only once women and children began to fall ill, along with recipients of infected blood products, straight men and injecting drug users that those responsible for protecting public health woke up.

Randy Shilts, in 1987 in *And the Band Played On*, painted a comprehensive picture of the evolution of the pandemic among gays, with tentative links to its origins in sub-Saharan Africa, and of which he was to die as one of its victims in 1994. But it was Peter Piot, who was later to become the Dean of the London school of Hygiene and Tropical Medicine, who filled in many of the gaps in his account of the virus's spread through Africa and out into the world. A laboratory medic with a fascination for both field work and anthropology, Piot found himself working as a young Belgian doctor in the 1970's in the Belgian Congo area of Africa, researching the exotic viruses that are responsible for the highly contagious and deadly haemorrhagic fevers.

If serendipity favours the prepared mind, he was most fortunate to find himself among a group that would throw light not only on HIV but also on the Ebola virus, which was to cause a major global public-health emergency almost 40 years later. In his account of his work in Africa, *No Time to Lose*, Piot describes the conditions under which it seems that some of these novel viruses emerge in human populations, having jumped species.

Centuries ago, outbreaks of viruses could take off like wild fire when previously unexposed humans would encounter a new culture, as happened with measles and the Pacific Islanders. The preconditions, however, for this to happen in our time appear to be where rapid urbanisation and sprawling slum settlements bring poverty-stricken and undernourished people into intimate contact with animals that may be harbouring commensal organisms. The animals themselves may be long adapted by evolution to these organisms, but they turn out to be pathogens for humans.

In the case of HIV and Ebola theories for these unknown viruses jumping species (the so-called zoonoses), include their ingestion in food through 'jungle meat' of one kind and another, perhaps monkeys or bats. In the case of HIV, Piot makes the argument that, once the virus had made its appearance in humans, its prevalence was amplified through the re-use of contaminated syringes by nursing nuns in a maternity unit; once it had infected poor women, some of whom were actively working in the sex industry and plying their trade among the truck drivers along the highway south to the mining regions and the miners of Southern Africa, the virus was well on its way to becoming a sexually transmitted disease.

When HIV arrived in the United Kingdom around 1984 it was in the middle of an epidemic of heroin injection among young people unable to find work. It took a Chief Medical Officer of an exceptional calibre, Sir Donald Acheson, to look beyond the social red-herrings. He prevented the slow-motion public-health car-crash by giving active support to local initiatives organised by individual public-health authorities in Liverpool and elsewhere.

The Irish-born Sir Donald Acheson was a clinical epidemiologist with an impressive track record of ground-breaking research into cancer of the nasal sinuses in woodworkers and the incrimination of blue asbestos into the crippling and fatal disease of asbestosis. Having established the new medical school in Southampton in 1970 as its inaugural Dean, his appointment as England's Chief Medical Officer in 1984 presented him with a set of enormous challenges.

His 1988 Report into the Salmonella and Legionnaires-disease failings at Stanley Royd psychogeriatric and at Stafford hospitals was a wake-up call for public health. Sir Donald next dealt with the pandemic of HIV/Aids and the fallout from BSE and proved adept at navigating the minefield that is the interface between national-level politics, academia and the nitty gritty realities of making a difference to public health at the front line. He has since been described aptly as 'the right man in the right place at the right time'.

As a politically savvy Chief Medical Officer with a strong humanitarian instinct, Sir Donald Acheson was able to navigate the increasingly puritanical Thatcher government and lend support to the first large-scale syringe exchange programme in the world, in Liverpool, which was experiencing particularly high levels of youth unemployment. Not only did this head off an epidemic of HIV infection in the Liverpool region, but, as an approach that came to be known as 'harm reduction', and as the 'Slow Burn' became a 'Rising Tide', this approach saved untold numbers of lives.

According to the book of Leviticus, in the Old Testament, it is not allowed to eat fallen stock, that is to say animals that have died from natural causes, but it is permissible to sell the meat from it to the next village. Failure to observe this law and the recycling of animal carcasses in animal feedstuffs was the cause of the BSE epidemic that began in the UK around 1986. This was in defiance of the fundamental precautionary principle that is the basis of public health and the practice of medicine to 'at least do no harm'. Caused by a primitive infectious agent composed of a protein that triggers the production of abnormal proteins in the brain, BSE is one of the causes of Creutzfeldt-Jakob disease which leads to progressive neurological deterioration, dementia and death.

A reluctance to recognise the reality of the emerging epidemic by British politicians because of its potential impact on the agricultural economy led to a delay in blowing the whistle, with the Minister of Agriculture of the time, John Gummer, seeking to reassure the public by holding a press conference in which his daughter publicly ate a beef burger. By the time systematic action was taken, with the removal of affected cattle from the food chain, the epidemic had become an international scandal with thousands of cases and around 200 deaths. Gummer's daughter's friend was among those who subsequently died of the disease. The cost of the BSE crisis is estimated at around £90 billion Europe-wide.

The outbreak of Hong Kong or Bird 'flu, came to public attention in May 1997 when a health worker who had been in contact with a boy who had died from the virus became ill-with a respiratory condition. It turned out that the boy had contracted the infection from poultry in one of Hong Kong's 'wet markets'. Animals are kept in often poor sanitary and overcrowded conditions, having been brought into the Special Administrative Region (SAR) of Hong Kong from peasant farms in mainland China to be sold live for the dinner table. By December, six months later, the cross-species infection from fowl to humans was confirmed with over 30 cases and four deaths, but at that time no examples of person-to-person transmission.

With concern about the potential for the virus to mutate and cause a human pandemic and with the daily import of 75,000 chickens from China, a drastic decision had to be taken. On a Sunday evening, with the eyes of the world on her, the Medical Officer of Health for Hong Kong, Margaret Chan, took the decision to have the entire Hong Kong poultry flock of over one million birds slaughtered. This prompt action ended the emergency but was an indication of what was coming over the next few years.

It proved to be another 'Slow-Burn' emergency, but it came with a tail. The next respiratory virus with the apparent potential to cause a pandemic was SARS-CoV, a close relative of COVID-19, in 2002, in the Guangdong province of China. This outbreak of SARS went on to cause almost 800 deaths from 8,000 cases in 37 countries until it petered out in July 2003. The failure to notify WHO led to an international row which has had resonances during the COVID-19 pandemic.

Just before Christmas, we were on a visit to China at the time and came across a small circulation English language newspaper in the hotel lobby in Beijing carrying a report of the first few cases. At the time no word of the outbreak had been reported outside China and recognising that this could be of some importance we faxed the relevant pages back to the public-health department at home to alert them to the news. The Chinese were slow in notifying the World Health Organization about what was happening and failed to do so until February 2003, over two months later. It turned out later that our fax had never been sent despite the assurances of the hotel staff in China that it had gone through.

In April 2009, seven years after the SARS epidemic, a pandemic of influenza broke out among pigs in Mexico, having seemingly come from the recombination of viruses passing between birds, swine and humans. This outbreak led to around 17,000 deaths worldwide and aroused high levels of concern internationally among a public increasingly sensitised to the idea that another, even on a par with 1918, could be on its way. Once person-to-person transmission had occurred, the Director General of the World Health Organization, who was by now the former Medical Officer for Health for Hong Kong, Margaret Chan, declared a Global Public Health Emergency.

This was the first time that such a thing had been called by WHO and when the pandemic tailed off that November it was followed by recriminations from those who claimed that the emergency had been called too soon. This dilemma of the threshold of when and if to invoke global measures to counteract epidemic emergencies has become a recurring theme in subsequent events.

When Ebola emerged in April 2014 as an epidemic emergency in West Africa and in Sierra Leone, where the UK had historic links, some, such as Peter Piot, who had been involved in identifying the virus many years before, were not surprised. Here was a highly contagious virus with a mortality rate of at least 50% that had turned up in a poverty stricken and remote part of the world affecting powerless people. But there had been little interest in researching the virus or exploring the possibilities of developing a vaccine when financial returns to pharmaceutical companies would be so unlikely. As with HIV/AIDS it was only when infections began to occur among people from the developed countries that the rest of the world paid attention, and even here it was slow off the mark. Several months were lost between April and August when finally a galvanised response began to appear.

Perhaps chastened by criticism of having overreacted with Swine 'flu in 2009, the WHO was reluctant and slow to act. The initial response was itself too narrowly focussed on the virology and medical aspects of the emergency. An early public-health focus came to be on the traditional burial practices involving intimate body washing rituals. It soon transpired that those involved, together with clinical workers who were brought in close contact with affected patients, were most likely to contract the virus and to die.

Unfortunately a mechanistic, male-centred analysis led to efforts at influencing burial practices through the authority of traditional, male, village chiefs. It was only when anthropologists became involved during the summer that it became clear that the centre of power over such matters, and any changes to be made, lay with the village women's committees. This then finally led to effective intervention.

This narrow drawing down of expertise would later become important in the British response to COVID-19 in 2020. It may be possible to escape mortality and economic disaster if only one or two factors converge to undermine a combative public-health response to a looming epidemic. But the accumulation of four, five, or more brings with it a sense of the inevitable.

Ironically, given the whole series of novel outbreaks of

infectious diseases that occurred in the years preceding COVID, it was probably the terrorist attacks on the World Trade Center in New York on September 11 2001 that had the unintended consequence of strengthening the world's capability for international public-health emergency measures. A subsequent spate of 'white powder' and anthrax scare incidents provided the added potential of bioterrorist attacks.

The fear of what our fellow humans might do, raised public health as a key security objective. What had merely been the tail-end of the highly secretive remnants of Cold War planning received a seat at the main table. In the UK, for example, planning for such threats had until 2001 been predominantly the province of the military and special intelligence agencies together with the police.

One outcome in England was the abolition in 2003 of the Health Education Authority and its replacement by the Health Protection Agency. It brought together the Public Health Laboratory Service and its national and regional laboratories with the top secret biological and chemical weapons laboratories in Porton Down and other aspects of toxicology and nuclear radiation that might constitute threats to public health. The latter would, for example, expertly trace the rare poisons used to attack former secret agents Alexander Litvinenko and Sergei Skripal on British soil to Russia. With this renewed focus on public health the next few years were something of a golden period. Previous governments' Cinderella, the British public-health system, suddenly had access, too, to state of the art science and protocols when combatting epidemics caused by pathogens. The response to a threat like COVID would now be as swift and as decisive as if a team of foreign spies were creating havoc in the country.

Given the public-health revival, where did it all go so wrong with COVID-19?

3

A Disaster Waiting to Happen

The experiences from almost two centuries of public health in Britain are object lessons of the fact that a rapid response against a novel pathogen attack with minimal economic costs only has a chance if decisions are left to local experts. In such battles the main heroes are local ones who understand exactly the habits and issues in their area. They can develop effective initiatives and formulate the tools they need to combat the spread of the pathogen in their area. A one-size fits all top-down response will simply not be as effective in containing a pathogen.

The 2018 *novichok* poisoning of Sergei Skripal and his daughter in Salisbury illustrate this lesson potently in the case of an attack organised by humans. All Tracy Daskiewicz, the Wiltshire Director of Public Health, knew was that two people collapsed on a bench for no apparent reason. She immediately understood the public-health implications of this unspecified risk and set about contact-tracing anyone near the couple, despite incredulity of the police, and to establish a web of containment. This soon included sealing off Salisbury—against strong business opposition—until the nature of the pathogen was established. After *novichok* was identified at Porton Down laboratory, and the manner of its extreme toxicity no longer a mystery, it became clear that her prompt decisions on the ground had saved hundreds from death and disability, caused by the minute quantity of the chemical toxin even though, tragically, one Salisbury resident, Dawn Sturgess, did die as a result of Russia's plot.

Many of the public-health improvements in Britain followed the appointment of Liam Donaldson as successor to Sir Donald Acheson as Chief Medical Officer. Donaldson was the first Chief Medical Officer to have completed a full five-year postgraduate training in public health and had since held senior posts in the North East of England where he combined the position of Regional Director of Public Health with that of Chief Executive of the NHS in the region. Although notionally the position of Chief Medical Officer for England complements those of the Chief Medical Officers for Scotland, Wales and Northern Ireland, the post holder is in reality the overarching Chief Medical Officer to the government in Whitehall and to the UK prime minister.

In addition, the new government, elected in the 1997 general election, had already committed itself to developing public health through the appointment of the country's first Minister for Public Health, the highly regarded Tessa Jowell, an MP with a background in social work and mental health. A Public Health White Paper followed in 1999 and from it flowed a series of initiatives aimed at tackling the growing inequalities in health that had become worse over the previous 20 years and the narrow focus on biological and medical science as the sole solution to issues of public health.

These initiatives included the Sure Start programme, together with the creation of Sure Start Centres based on John F. Kennedy's 'Head Start' initiative as US President. The centres provided parental support and childhood enrichment for the 20% most disadvantaged children, together with Health Action Zones and Healthy Living Centres.

Liam Donaldson, furthermore, set about building a strong set of national and regional public-health arrangements by mobilising the nine Regional Directors as a national team of experts. They provided day-to-day strategic leadership to the on-the-ground, local public-health system by working with local public-health directors. But they also each held responsibilities at the national level. Each one of the nine had a different government department to provide input to. This created an adaptable matrix through which local, regional and national information flowed efficiently and freely without the usual, centralised fits and starts of Whitehall turf wars and compartmentalisation, or other Westminster-centric control and data-hogging issues. N

At the local level the career structure for public health took an imaginative leap with the opening up of opportunities for those who had been training in the discipline from non-medical backgrounds. During this period many of them became Directors of Public Health in what had previously been a narrowly medically-defined enterprise.

The fallout from the September 11 atrocity in New York resulted in a Civil Contingency Act of Parliament in 2004 which created a coherent structure for emergency planning on the ground throughout Britain. A clear set of roles and responsibilities were established for those involved in emergency preparation and response at the local level. This included tasking emergency services, local authorities and NHS organisations to prepare for adverse events and incidents through the preparation and exercising of emergency plans and the identification of lead or so-called 'Category 1 responders'. One specific aspect of the new legislation was the identification of local Directors of Public Health as having lead roles in the event of bio-terrorist incidents that required specialised bio-medical input.

The remaining years of the decade were characterised by a continuing emphasis on health-emergency planning with regular 'table-top' and real-time exercises. Following the 2009 Swine 'flu pandemic, a review in 2010 of the performance of the national public-health response carried out by the former Chief Medical

Officer for Wales, Dame Deirdre Hine, concluded that the system had performed well. As a result of the report, and its recommendations for further improvements, significant additional investment was made. This included supplies such as Personal Protective Equipment (PPE) for front line staff.

Austerity strikes

While initially much of the emergency planning was centred on the need to be prepared for terrorist attacks that might include biological or nuclear components, concern about the possibilities of pandemic influenza were also very much in mind at this time, following the Avian 'flu of 1997 and then SARS in 2002.

This is reflected in the NHS and Cabinet Office planning guidance documents for pandemic influenza. These were produced and regularly updated until 2013. Hereafter these regular updates appear to have ended in England but not in Scotland. For example, NHS Highland produced a contingency plan for pandemic Influenza dated 29 December 2016. In the same year, even in England a major influenza planning exercise, 'Operation Cygnus', was held.

In understanding why there was this neglect of health emergency planning during these years several significant factors were of importance.

The global economic turmoil that began in 2008 combined with a change in government at Westminster in 2010 to reduce the finances available for all public services including public health.

However it is likely that of greater importance was the wholesale reorganisation of both the National Health Service and the arrangements for public health by then health secretary Andrew Lansley. These fractured a system that had performed well. The NHS Chief Executive of the time, Sir David Nicholson, described it as 'So big you could see it from space'. The net result was that the reorganisation did away with Donaldson's organisational structures and reverted to centralisation of public health, bringing public health back under a London cosh.

Public health directors and their teams were relocated from the National Health Service back into local authorities, from which they had come 40 years before. A new national public-health agency, Public Health England, was created with its headquarters close to Whitehall. The nine regional directors of public health were reduced to four who were closely accountable to ministers.

Although welcomed by many, the move of local public-health directors back into the town hall was not universally popular. The theory was that this location might provide better opportunities for public-health teams to influence local government. One consequence was the weakening of the links between public health and the clinical world of the NHS.

The downside rapidly became apparent. Local government had changed a great deal since 1974. Councils had become management offices. Many of the historic functions relevant to public health had been removed, long since privatised, or transformed into arm's length organisations: municipal housing, water and sewerage, street cleansing, police constabularies, fire and rescue, recreation facilities and local schools, among others.

One consequence of this was that many local directors of public health found themselves to be heading up small teams that continued to shrink as their budgets were progressively cut under the austerity regime imposed from London, something that the directors at Public Health England weren't able to or didn't resist in a bid not to challenge new budgets set by Whitehall.

In a bitter irony public-health directors now found their status downgraded to one in which they were frequently line-managed by the local director of adult social care. They lost their automatic, direct access to either the local authority chief executive or the leader of the council and had to wait for their adult-social-care line manager to allow them such access.

41

This situation was a consequence of the arcane practise whereby the job weight of a director was calculated. Status and salary in the civil service and local government was arrived at by reference to the size of the senior officer's budgetary responsibility and the numbers of line-managed staff. The loss of public-health budget meant also loss of independence—an intended or unintended consequence of the cuts depending on which way you look at Whitehall internecine wars. What certainly was irrelevant to the new local-government organograms was the skill-set necessary to influence all agencies and bodies across a local government area and to ensure that the population's health is protected.

By 2013, by and large, this development was complete. Directors of adult social care were the only officers left with a large budget and large numbers of staff and so became second in importance only to the chief executive of local councils. The critical ability for local public-health directors to be able to 'command a room or a meeting' and to influence and communicate across the whole borough and its stake holders had gone missing. Freedom of speech and action was curtailed, and that included the statutory duty to produce an independent annual public-health report. These reports with potentially embarrassing facts and figures were now safely cocooned within a superior structure where they could be managed. Links with clinicians and clinical services in the NHS were weakened, if only because there was no staff left to cover the distance in regular meetings.

Nationally there was criticism of Public Health England, not least by the Health Select Committee under the chairmanship of Conservative MP, Sarah Wollaston. Many believed that it was neither fish nor fowl, both too close to government to offer a critical voice nor close enough to be influential. At the same time, under a new Chief Medical Officer for England, Sally Davies, a research-clinician by training, the public-health expertise available to ministers in the Department of Health was both neglected and run down. These chickens were destined to come home to roost with a vengeance when COVID struck.

Pandemic 'flu planning—taking eyes off the ball
Even though the 139 local public-health directors had by 2020 been side-lined, and the regional level diminished, in theory they could still be activated in a crisis. Public Health England (PHE) could instruct them to join the front-line as PHE had done in Salisbury in 2018. It had provided the Wiltshire public-health team with the authority, and access to data, it needed to deal well with the disaster. Likewise, with its national purview, PHE could have provided cabinet ministers with detailed steers on the areas bearing the brunt of a pandemic from local data gathered by its directors if there had been adequate testing capacity.

However, in the case of COVID which threatened the whole of Britain, PHE acted very differently from when it was dealing with the isolated Skripal-*novichok* spy crisis in Salisbury. PHE withheld the early information it received on the virus from its own local directors. Furthermore, it even refused to release all available data on the virus, including test results, if a local-director specifically asked for it. In what must one of the most egregious scandals of public health, this stone-walling of its own staff on the ground continued for the duration of the lockdown. PHE only started sharing postcode data on test results, an essential piece of information, with its directors and local authorities on 1 July, three days before the end of the lockdown, through a digital dashboard. It was as if the Battle of Britain was about to be fought with RAF pilots who were given neither information about enemy planes, nor ammunition, nor even accurate radar information where attacks were happening and weren't even allowed to go to their planes.

What PHE did do was instruct its staff under no circum-stances to talk to the media without authorisation from PHE or their local-government line manager. If *novichok* had been handled like COVID, people might still be dying from the toxin and parts of the Salisbury economy might still unnecessarily be in lockdown. The Wiltshire director of public health would meanwhile be sitting in her office trying to get information from PHE while declining calls from the media.

How did this inexplicable situation come about? The minister in charge of PHE was Johnson's health minister Matt Hancock. Reasonably, one should ask what decisions did the health minister make?

The assumptions made in the British Cabinet Office 'Preparing for Pandemic Influenza, Guidance for Local Planners' (July 2013), would have made a useful starting point for a tailored COVID-19 response. Since it came from the cabinet office, it would even have helped Boris Johnson himself. It would have helped minimise the pandemic's health impact and pushed Britain towards the top of the global list of countries that both weathered the storm in mortality, social and economic upheaval.

The underlying assumption underpinning that guidance was of 'the rapid spread of (influenza) caused by a novel virus strain to which people would have no immunity resulting in more serious illness than caused by seasonal influenza'. Under such cir-cumstances the guidance stated that the strategic objectives would be to minimise the health impacts by supporting interna-tional efforts to detect its emergence, and early assessment of the virus by sharing scientific information; promoting individual responsibility and action to reduce the spread of infection through good hygiene practices.

Notably it didn't have a narrow NHS focus, such as might prevail while acting in a panic without a plan. The guidance ensured that social-care systems were also ready to provide treatment and support for the large numbers likely to suffer. The guidance, furthermore, addressed the fact that an emergency response would have a knock-on effect on all public services and that this would create its own havoc and exacerbate the effects of a pandemic. Thus, it framed a response that would ensure that all other essential care would continue unaffected rather than deteriorate and turn those reliant on it into prey for the pandemic.

In addition, the guidance went even further. It addressed the wider impact of a pandemic on society and the economy by supporting the continuity of essential services, including the supply of essential medicines and protecting essential national infrastructure as far as possible; supporting the continuation of everyday activities as far as practicable; and preparing to cope with the possibility of significant numbers of additional deaths whilst promoting a return to normality and the restoration of disrupted services at the earliest opportunity.

Finally, there were the hearts and minds—one of the most significant issues in terms of what was to come with COVID-19. The guidance set out the importance of instilling and maintaining trust and confidence by 'ensuring that health and other professionals, the public and the media are engaged and well-informed in advance of and throughout the pandemic period and that health and other professionals receive information and guidance in a timely way so they can respond to the public appropriately'.

Failure to adhere to what was set out in the 2013 Cabinet Office guidance would prove to be fatal in 2020.

One of the criticisms that would later be made of the UK government's preparedness for the COVID pandemic was that it was too heavily dependent on models for dealing with Influenza. Whilst this may have been true when it came to the specifics—not least with the arguments that would occur over testing and tracing for the virus—there were many other protocols from the earlier planning documents that would have put the UK in a much better place to act effectively. Instead there continues to be a power vacuum in Whitehall that sucks the air out of a concerted public-health effort for Britain.

COVID-19 is not a virus similar to the Influenza of 1919, but is related to the SARS virus of 2003. This has implications in key aspects of its public-health management. Nonetheless, the assumptions put forward in planning for a viral pandemic had relevance. The guidance hypothesised that from the first arrival of the virus in the country it would probably be a further week or two before there were sporadic cases across the country. A pandemic may occur in one wave or a series of waves lasting 12-15 weeks. These may occur after the pandemic appears to be over and may be more severe than earlier waves. A worst case of a 50% clinical-attack rate of symptoms, ranging from mild to severe with hospitalisation rates of 1-4% of those showing symptoms, was postulated. It assumed different areas would be under pressure at different times and that the death rate could be of the order of 2.5%. It had modelled for staff absenteeism of 15-20% during the peak weeks as a result of the measures in the guidance and set up a plan to liaise with the business community to minimise disruption.

One could argue that a plan dating back seven years to 2013 is an eternity in political terms for any government. But can the same be said for the year 2016? What if Whitehall and the government knew in that year that it was found wanting on all those points?

When the COVID-19 pandemic gathered momentum in March and April 2020, word got out about Exercise Cygnus that had taken place in October 2016 in England. It was the table-top training simulation of a pandemic caused by an unknown virulent Influenza strain. This had been shortly after the referendum on 26 July that would sweep the country out of the European Union and Boris Johnson into the cabinet as Foreign Secretary.

Cited in the *New Statesman* on her part in Cygnus, Chief Medical Officer Dame Sally Davies observed that 'We've just had in the UK a three-day exercise on 'flu in a pandemic that killed a lot of people. It became clear that we could not cope with the excess bodies'. One lethal issue, according to Davies, was that Britain faced the threat of 'inadequate ventilation' where people suffered from Respiratory Distress Syndrome resulting from infection. A full report on the exercise was produced in 2017. But it was never published, never acted on, and disappeared in a Whitehall drawer for being inconvenient in the way critical reports always are—unless they are neutral or positive, in which case they're put on a shelf.

With mounting pressure on Boris Johnson's government, which refused to release it, the report was leaked to the *Guardian* newspaper who published its main findings on May 7, 2020.

According to the newspaper, Exercise Cygnus was a simulation in which participants were invited to imagine that they were fighting a fictitious 'worst-case-scenario' 'flu pandemic affecting 50% of the population and causing up to 400,000 excess deaths.

The scenario considered the situation involving a novel virus that had emerged from Thailand and that later transpired to be an H2N2 strain of influenza, originating in swans. The World Health Organization declared a Public Health Emergency four weeks into the outbreak, triggering the UK response at a national level. Over the three days of the UK exercise, participants role-played the emergency response in the seventh week of the pandemic when they might be faced with extreme demands on medical and social care. Mock COBR (popularly known as COBRA—the A standing for room A) meetings were held while simulations included those of mainstream media responses.

According to the scathing, unpublished Cygnus report, 'The UK's preparedness and response, in terms of its plans, policies and capability, is currently not sufficient to cope with the extreme demands of a severe pandemic that will have a nationwide impact across all sectors'.

Other findings included a lack of joining up and of tactical plans between pandemic responses and procedures, with plans that were severely out of date and were relying on organisational memory of fighting the 2009 Swine 'flu pandemic, since when there had been wholesale structural reorganisation of health services and of public health.

Particular concern was expressed about the lack of capacity in the fragmented social care sector which was almost entirely privately run by a plethora of providers.

The report offered an extensive list of lessons learned and recommendations, very few of which seem to have been implemented or followed through, although in a media interview in March 2020, health secretary Matt Hancock denied these claims.

The curious thing, however, is that half of the failures of Britain's COVID response were carbon copies of the issues raised in the report, as we will see. Matt Hancock's denial was one more in what would become a very long line of denials the government would issue. It was an early indication that the Johnson cabinet lacked a basic understanding of the role of government in a crisis, remained and remains disorganised, and was far more interested in slapping down dissent from London than in devising a strategy that with military precision maximised the attack against the virus while neutralising its knock-on effect on social services and damage to the economy at large.

In July, the ONS published Britain's excess death figures covering the lockdown. They were arrived at by taking the actual deaths during the lockdown and deducting the statistical average mortality for these months calculated over the previous five years. Thus the excess-death figures included both deaths where the death certificate cited COVID and those resulting in an unspecified way from COVID measures, delayed operations, etc. According to some there were months with more than twice as many deaths as normal. Britain, under Boris Johnson's government, scored the highest number of excess deaths of all European countries during the first five months of the pandemic.

4

A Rising Tide in Wuhan, China

On 5 January 2020 the World Health Organization reported that on 31 December 2019 its office in China had been informed by the national authorities that cases of pneumonia of unknown cause had been occurring in Wuhan city in the Hubei Province. As of 3 January, 44 patients had been reported, of whom 11 were severely ill. Some of the patients had been workers in the Huanon Seafood market and on 1 January the seafood market was closed for environmental sanitation and disinfection. Later China was to ban the trade of live animals at wet markets together with the buying, selling and transportation of wild animals in markets, restaurants and online marketplaces.

Although the causal agent had not been identified early suggestions were that a novel virus had jumped species from pangolins or bats, both regarded as delicacies in China. There were also a spate of conspiracy theories that a new virus had been developed in a local laboratory in Wuhan and had escaped. On 7 January the Chinese authorities identified the pathogen responsible for the infections as a new type of coronavirus, similar to the SARS virus of 2002-3 and belonging to the same group of viruses as the common cold and epidemic viral pneumonia. The same day China shared the genetic code of the new virus which would later be named COVID-19 by WHO to distinguish it from other coronaviruses.

At that stage 121 close contacts had been identified and placed under medical observation with follow up whilst investigations were carried out into the underlying cause along with active case finding and retrospective investigation. Based on the information provided by the Chinese authorities WHO's recommendations were that the public-health measures applicable to influenza and severe acute respiratory infections should still apply; that no specific measures were necessary for travellers but that should travellers returning from the area develop symptoms suggestive of respiratory illness they should seek medical attention and share their travel history. WHO's advice against the application of travel or trade restrictions with China would subsequently become contentious with allegations that they had pulled their punches for reasons of diplomacy.

Early accounts of the illness caused by COVID-19 described a 'flu-like illness characterised by cough, runny nose, sore throat, high temperature and shortness of breath proceeding in a proportion of people to pneumonia requiring the intervention with penetrative ventilation. As knowledge was acquired with increasing numbers of cases this picture would turn out to be incomplete, especially with regard to the extent of multiple organ involvement and the value of radical ventilation procedures.

Not surprisingly, in view of China's history of being slow to inform the international community of previous novel outbreaks, such as SARS in 2002, this would also become a contested issue, particularly in the US. President Donald Trump, began to refer to the new virus as 'The Chinese Virus'. Suggestions were made that the Wuhan epidemic may in fact have occurred much earlier together with later reports, contested by China, that satellite images indicated increases in hospital traffic from the previous autumn onwards. Considering my first-hand experience with the mysteriously un-sent SARS fax I dispatched from Beijing in

December 2002, it is hard not to trust the satellite images more than the denials from China's one-party government.

The battle to control the emerging narrative took a dark turn with the tragic story of Wuhan ophthalmologist and whistle blower, 33-year-old Li Wenliang. This young medical consultant had sent a warning to colleagues on 30 December reporting to them about seven cases of patients he had seen with a virus that he thought looked like SARS. Days later he was summoned to the Police Security Bureau in which he was accused of making false comments and 'severely disturbing the social order' as one of eight people accused of spreading rumours. Dr Li developed symptoms of the illness himself on 10 January, was diagnosed with COVID-19 on 30 January and his death was announced on 7 February.

Li's death led to an outpouring of anger and grief in China creating a crisis for the Chinese government that seemed to bring about a change in attitude with much closer involvement of the World Health Organization in overseeing the collation and publication of data about the numbers of cases and deaths.

As January progressed so did disturbing reports in mainstream and social media about exponentially increasing numbers of deaths in Wuhan. The first death was reported on 11 January, a 61-year-old man who had been a regular customer at the seafood market in Wuhan. This death occurred shortly before the major Chinese holiday period of Chinese New Year, which is characterised by massive movements of people across the country with millions of urban workers returning to their families in their home villages.

On 13 January the first confirmed case outside China was diagnosed, that of a 61-year-old woman in Thailand, who had been in Wuhan. Airports in south-east Asia promptly began to screen passengers for fever. As the numbers of those confirmed to be infected in Wuhan reached 282, cases began to occur in Japan, South Korea and the US. They were all visitors to Wuhan.

On 21 January, with 500 global infections, the China health ministry finally confirmed that human to human transmission of the SARS-like virus was occurring. Wuhan, a city of 11 million people, was cut off on 23 January by the Chinese authorities. It was followed by the lockdown of the 60-million population of Hubei province, constituting the largest quarantine in human history. All transport in and out of the province was stopped, shops, schools and universities were closed, public transport suspended and private vehicles severely restricted.

By the time off this lockdown the numbers of cases worldwide was doubling every 1-3 days and by 31 January there had been a reported 258 deaths in China. The numbers reported by China were to be revised sharply upwards in April when, in response to criticism of the country's lack of transparency, the World Health Organization became involved in validating the diagnostic data. The 50% increase in the numbers reported at that time, with a national total of 4,636 deaths, according to Johns Hopkins University, was explained by the inclusion of deaths that had occurred outside of hospitals.

Later a modelling exercise by the highly regarded Rand Corporation, based on air passenger movements and the international spread of the virus, would conclude that the likely number of cases in China could have been 37 times higher than the daily average of 172 reported between 31 December and 22 January. This issue of the discrepancies between government-reported cases and deaths was also to become a major one at the height of the pandemic in the UK under Boris Johnson's recently elected government.

On 24 January the first scientific paper on the epidemic was published in *The Lancet* by a group of Chinese clinicians and researchers reporting that one third of those patients admitted to hospital required intensive care with one-third of them requiring ventilation. According to the *Guardian* newspaper, following a meeting of the government's emergency committee, COBR, the UK health secretary Matt Hancock stated that the risk to the public remained low. With the benefit of now knowing some of the information available to Johnson's cabinet, it is not easy to see how the minister was able to deny the gravity of the situation.

Professor Neil Ferguson, a statistical modeller from London's Imperial College, advised ministers and officials that the infectivity rate of the new virus (R0), was between 2.6 and 3.5, compared with the Spanish 'flu rate of between 2.0 and 3.0 and that it would require a 60% reduction in transmission to get on top of it; advice that was underlined by a note from the New England Complex Systems Institute on 26 January of the necessity to act swiftly.

On 30 January the World Health Organization declared that the coronavirus outbreak was a 'Public Health Emergency of International Concern' (PHEIC). In response UK government raised the threat level from low to moderate.

The following day, 31 January, the UK parliament finally passed the legislation to leave the European Union. This was to prove significant.

5

The Virus Arrives in the UK

In mid-January, as cases of the new coronavirus infection began to be reported from around the world, the World Health Organization had stated that it was too early to declare an international public-health emergency. Speaking on 23 January, Dr Tedros Adhanom Ghebreyesus, the Director General of WHO, said at the time that 'it has not yet become a global health emergency but it may become one'. He went on to say that 'we know that most of those who have died had underlying health conditions such as hypertension, diabetes, or cardiovascular disease, that weakened their immune systems' and that although there was human to human transmission in China there was no evidence of it elsewhere at that time, admitting that there was still a great deal that was unknown about the virus, how easily it was spread, its clinical course and severity.

For Peter Piot, whose work on the HIV and Ebola viruses in the 1970's and 80's had made him a foremost authority on novel viruses there were 'still many missing pieces in the jigsaw puzzle'. He predicted that 'over the coming days and weeks we will know much more, but there cannot be any complacency as to the need for global action', whilst observing that 'the good news is that the data to date suggest that this virus may have a lower mortality rate than SARS, we have a diagnostic test and there is greater transparency than decades gone by'.

Sadly Piot—who was to become infected with the virus himself but fortunately made a recovery—was being optimistic about some governments' commitment to transparency and ability to deliver on large scale testing. Certainly Johnson's cabinet would rank closely with the Chinese government on the former.

By this time concern was beginning to grow in the UK media with a spate of news stories appearing in the media the same day as Dr Tedros's tentative announcement. On the same day, the Press Association drew attention to 14 people having been tested in the UK. Five came back negative, whilst results were awaited on the remaining nine. Two people being tested in Scotland were diagnosed with Influenza, having returned from Wuhan, in China.

Among the most interesting was the Sky News report on the experience of one British man, Craig Dillon, who had returned home from holiday in Australia, via China, and had developed 'flu symptoms. Dillon said, 'I had been experiencing 'flu symptoms for about a week to two weeks.... [I] went to work early Wednesday, but I was still feeling 'flu-ey and it started to get worse and worse. I eventually called the NHS 111 number after feeling extremely ill and faint. They told me to go to hospital immediately.'

The unusual treatment he received at the hospital made the story with hindsight an anatomy of the COVID response in Johnson's cabinet in January. Dillon continued, 'When I got to St Thomas's I went to A&E and told them my symptoms and that I had been to China and Thailand. The doctor literally dragged me outside the hospital near the ambulance bay and put a mask on me... then a nurse and doctor came in full hazmat suits... they ran multiple blood tests, mouth swabs and nose swabs... had to wait until the results came back.' Evidently, the NHS grapevine connecting its million-plus staff members was on high alert about the appearance of an unknown Coronavirus, even as the health minister himself in private denied reportedly that it was anything but a low risk.

Craig Dillon as a person was interesting, too. The twenty-seven-year old was no ordinary traveller. He was the founder of social media agency Westminster Digital and had advised Boris Johnson on his leadership campaign and in the general election. In fact, he had also advised executive cabinet minister Michael Gove and Johnson's two most senior cabinet ministers, Dominic Raab and Sajid Javid, who was then still Chancellor of the Exchequer.

As a result of his A&E visit, Dillon, unlike Britain's health minister Hancock ostensibly, straightaway got Britain's brewing disaster. He told Sky News, 'Luckily, my results were negative and I probably didn't have coronavirus.... the problem is that I landed at Heathrow and met all my friends and went to work and to Starbucks. There should have been something more at Heathrow that could detect my temperature was really high—but I guess we don't have that technology yet.' It probably wasn't a coincidence, but that same day the government announced that something was being organised at Heathrow, the airport where Dillon had flown in. Grant Shapps, Johnson's Transport Secretary, the number sixteen in the Cabinet, announced a few hours later on Sky News that a 'separate area' was being set up. The reason given was 'as airports around the world step up screening of travellers from affected regions at the centre of the coronavirus outbreak.'

This *ad-hoc* Heathrow area was later to become a mystery in its own right. Unless it wasn't a coincidence after all and seeing one of its own key spin-doctors on TV had spurred someone in the government to cover the media 'problem' with Heathrow in case it might inconveniently boomerang in the news at a later stage. Why would the Johnson government only address direct flights from China to Heathrow, but were screening arrangements not rolled out to all other air and sea ports of entry into the UK? Obviously Westminster did not seriously think that the virus would choose to piggy-back only on travellers flying straight in from Wuhan. (Or did it?) Nor were the *ad-hoc* screening arrangements at Heathrow themselves anything but off-hand. They were far less comprehensive than those adopted by countries that would be much more successful in containing the virus at this critical early stage.

The Hillingdon Director of Public Health, under which Heathrow falls, and all the directors of other ports of entry would have had very different ideas about this. That is, if they had been involved from the start like the Wiltshire Public Health Director in the Skripal case. They would have been on it from the first WHO communications about the new virus, if not from the even earlier reports in the media. As it was, they were out of the loop and powerless to act *ex-officio* in any case.

In the light of the uncertainties that have subsequently arisen about the sensitivity and specificity of tests for the coronavirus at the beginning of the outbreak, and in view of the nature and course of Mr Dillon's clinical symptoms, it must also remain an open question as to whether he was among the first cases in the country. Did he inadvertently contribute to the early seeding of the domestic epidemic? His closeness to Britain's top ministers, several of whom caught COVID-19, also begs the question whether he may have been patient zero to the highest echelon of London power when, as he told Sky News, he met friends and went to work before his visit to A&E.

It would was an ominous snap-shot of the re-elected cabinet in action. A twenty seven year old on the ground without medical training saw the threat, but his election clients Boris Johnson and his top cabinet, with all the facts at their fingertips and with wall-to-wall senior civil servants and advisors such as the Dominic Cummings, did not.

Mimicking China's approach, Public Health England (PHE) refused to give the media a breakdown of where the people had been tested and where the negative results were recorded. In fact, PHE was even more secretive than China as very few of its own 5,500 staff were given access to these details. The organisation was headed by Duncan Selbie, who reported directly to health secretary Matt Hancock. Like his counterparts in China, it seems Hancock wanted a hermetic seal on any information that could harm the government.

Selbie had been appointed in 2013 as PHE's first chief executive despite his lack of background in the area. He himself had joked when accepting the £185,000 a year job, 'you can fit my public-health credentials on a postage stamp'. The PHE's refusal to provide transparent data was an early public sign of the stone-walling that was to characterise the PHE's PR's approach on behalf of the Johnson government to the emergency.

With domestic concern mounting, the week of January 27 in the UK was not an auspicious one to be faced with a global public-health emergency. Over three years of political paralysis following the referendum committing the country to leave the European Union, the national drama was heading to some kind of conclusion. One of the main news items of the week was the argument about whether Big Ben at the House of Commons would be allowed to chime at the moment when, to protagonists of 'Brexit', the country would 'take back control'. A spirit of jingoism gripped many in the country.

Despite the fact that there was a dangerous new virus at large, that it was now fast spreading internationally, and that the World Health Organization was about to declare a Public Health Emergency of International Concern, this did not appear to be high in the government priorities. This should have been about to change.

During the course of the week things had begun to move quite fast behind the scenes as it became apparent that a large number of British citizens had been trapped in Wuhan by the lockdown in the city. To everybody's surprise there was an announcement out of the blue on the Wednesday afternoon, 30 January, that a plane load of evacuees would be on their way home. As reported in the *Liverpool Echo* that evening:

> Around 100 British nationals evacuated from the Chinese city at the centre of the coronavirus outbreak will be held in quarantine on Merseyside. The flight, set to leave Wuhan city tonight is expected to arrive at RAF airbase Brize Norton, in Oxfordshire, on Friday morning. They will then be transported to a former student accommodation block on the grounds of Arrowe Park hospital (on the Wirral). The *Echo* understands staff who lived there were given 12 hours to move out.

This news coincided with other news, reported the same day, that 'a man has been rushed to hospital in York after falling unwell'.

While noting that the coronavirus had at that time killed an estimated 170 people and spread to 15 countries since starting in China, the *Echo* quoted Foreign Secretary, Dominic Raab, as saying 'We've been working flat out, 24/7 [a phrase that was to become as common over the next four months as denials], to try and make sure we can identify British nationals in Wuhan, get them to a muster point and get them to a flight, a chartered flight in and out'. Passengers would be quarantined for a period of 14 days according to the Press Association.

The 83 evacuees from Wuhan arrived at Arrowe Park shortly after 19.15 on the Friday evening in a convoy of coaches from Brize Norton as the country prepared to leave the European Union at 23.00 that same day. At the same time it was now being reported that two Chinese nationals from the same family who had been staying at the Staycity apartment-hotel in York had tested positive for coronavirus and been taken to the infectious diseases unit at the Royal Victoria Infirmary in Newcastle upon Tyne. The virus had definitely now arrived in the UK.

Professor Chris Whitty, the recently appointed Chief Medical Officer for England as successor to Dame Sally Davies commented that the NHS was 'extremely well-prepared for managing infections and it was trying to identify any close contacts the two patients had to prevent further spread'. Professor Whitty said that the unit in Newcastle was experienced in treating people with infectious diseases, that there was a high chance that people would get better, and that a lot of people would end up with a relatively minor disease. He added, 'the small number who go on to be more seriously ill tend to develop respiratory problems which will be dealt with as anyone else with a respiratory disease'.

According to Public Health England (PHE) close contacts included 'anybody who was within two metres of the infected person for 15 minutes, that the virus could probably survive on a tissue for 15 minutes, but that it was unlikely to survive on door handles, for more than 24 hours'. PHE went on to claim that there was minimal risk to either guests or staff at the Staycity property in York, that those identified as close contacts would be given health advice about symptoms and an emergency number in case they became unwell, but wouldn't be quarantined. Professor Ian Jones, professor of virology at the University of Reading, said that the possibility of further spread was 'minimal' because the cases were caught early.

This would be the first of a series of advisory assurances given by authorities. But how these assurances could have been arrived at, apart from being wishful thinking, was difficult to see. While the new virus itself had been identified by China its virulence was not yet understood by anyone.

Those in the firing line didn't need to be told, however. The arrival of the Wuhan evacuees at Arrowe Park hospital, with no prior consultation and warning, prompted considerable community alarm and concern, not least with regard to the possibility of local community spread, and this resulted in a great deal of social media traffic and mainstream media interest.

It soon became apparent that communications concerning the developing emergency had not been thought through by PHE and other government officials, the cabinet included. It was the first crucial failure of the Johnson government, though how to avoid it was extensively highlighted by the 2013 cabinet guidance. No obvious single point of informed and trustworthy opinion was evident at the national level. At the local level there was silence from those who traditionally would have been the focal point for reliable information and public assurance, the local Directors of Public Health.

The Chief Medical Officer's statement in response to the cases in York was one of the few he was to make until mid-February but meanwhile there seemed to be a rush by ministers to be in the limelight and to own the publicity, at this point. Health secretary Matt Hancock vied with the transport secretary Grant Shapps, as did foreign secretary Dominic Raab and home secretary Priti Patel, the numbers three and four by seniority in the Johnson cabinet.

PHE, however, shone through its absence. It was the central vault where all the information in Britain regarding the virus came together so that it could be shared coherently, publicly and internally. But during the months of lockdown PHE was to respond to media requests for clarification only with the bare minimum. And what it did say tended to be soothing advice that turned out to be speculative, rather than an authoritative tally of what was by that time known about the virus. Wikipedia would have been a better source of information than PHE during the lockdown period.

It would be cynical to assume that cabinet ministers had started using PHE as their private piggy bank to plunder for information that would help them either manage the media narrative, or, more simply, muffle bad facts. But that is probably exactly how Whitehall saw PHE.

In the 2018 Skripal case, PHE had shown a similar pattern of secretive behaviour. The Skripals fell ill on 4 March and on the same day officers in Hazmat suits inspected the bench where they were found—not the normal response in the case of a 'drug overdose', the term used by officials. On 7 March it was made public that the cause was an as yet unnamed nerve agent. Despite the contact-tracing by the Wiltshire Public Health Director from day one, it nonetheless took PHE a whole week to issue advice to those who were at the same places as the Skripals to wash their clothes and possessions. Even this late advice hardly reflected the honest truth. The missing information hiding from this piece of public advice was how to cleanse a nerve agent in a manner that avoided contamination. Publicly, in a manner that governments in Beijing and Moscow wouldn't give a second thought, PHE treated potential contamination of the public at large as if it was but a patch of mud. Unlike Public Health Director Daszkiewicz, who was evidently on a chokehold media leash, PHE was taking a punt that further deaths would not occur.

As pandemic events came crashing down on the news wires, the mainstream media became increasingly exasperated at the difficulty in obtaining spokespeople at either national or local level. As a result, I soon found myself with regular requests for interviews as a public-health expert.

On the Saturday morning I received a request for a television interview from Sky News outside the quarantine building at Arrowe Park hospital and made the first of what would turn out to be many public-health analyses on national and local television, radio, print and new digital media as PHE remained silent. My approach to this was designed to inform the public what to expect without creating unnecessary alarm.

Sky News interview, 1 February
What we are seeing now are the first few cases in York and its

likely we will see more. With these situations it's like with the Millennial Bug when we took precautions coming up to the year 2000 with people concerned about computers crashing. We spent a lot of money and when it didn't happen people said 'what a waste of money!' You have to be prepared, to put the effort in, and then if it doesn't happen, great! People should be concerned, concerned in order to take action and to look after themselves.

As the weeks passed, and with them growing evidence of an inadequate government response, these interviews were to multiply as the media was desperate to have an authoritative perspective on the fast-developing news story.

Behind Whitehall walls, meanwhile the top of the civil service started buzzing to a different tune. When one of those quarantined at Arrowe Park threatened to abscond the government quietly passed an order in parliament giving it extra powers of detention under the Public Health (Control of Disease) Act, 1984, a piece of tidying up legislation that was little known. There was very little discussion about its contents or implications with just a note appearing on the government website on 10 February: 'In light of the recent public-health emergency from the novel Coronavirus originating from Wuhan, the Secretary of State has made regulations to ensure that the public are protected as far as possible from the transmission of the virus. In accordance with Regulation 3, the Secretary of State declares that the incidence or transmission of novel Coronavirus constitutes a serious and imminent threat to public health, and the measures outlined in these regulations are considered as an effective means of delaying or preventing further transmission of the virus'.

Likewise, there was what the intelligence services were told. Returning from an early-February COBR meeting with Whitty and chief scientific adviser Sir Patrick Vallance, head of MI5 Sir

Andrew Parker was warned about the impending pandemic. 'Having been told this is coming, pretty much that day I instructed the implementation of our contingency plan for pandemic 'flu', he let slip during a Royal Society of Medicine webinar in the last weeks of the lockdown. The probability, he was told at the COBR meeting, was 'high and strong'.

If any evidence was needed that the link between the security services and public health forged under Liam Donaldson had been severed this was it. In Salisbury, the security services had a one or two day head start on the public when they took over the crime scene. In the case of the pandemic, MI5 was notified a month and a half before the British public.

On his official blog, Head of PHE Duncan Selbie posted one of PHE's rare public statements on 21 February. The 139 words started with the sentence, 'There have been no new positive cases this week in the UK, which is testament to the robust infection control measures in place, as well as the diagnostic and testing work that is happening in laboratories across the country.' It was government cheer-leading masquerading as public information.

The guidance it linked to was withdrawn on 13 March, the day the government suddenly announced the lockdown, also straight from the big-brother handbook. During this period, PHE's local Directors of Public Health remained muzzled and were not given the information they asked for. The Battle of Britain was being fought without its pilots and relied solely on NHS staff on the ground and Whitehall in London to stem the attack. No one said it, but PHE's head office in London had become the government's good-news front.

6

News from Bahrain

An invitation to advise

The Kingdom of Bahrain is a sovereign state, made up of an archipelago of islands with the capital Manama occupying a strategic position on Bahrain Island in the Persian Gulf. Formerly a British Protectorate, the kingdom is a constitutional monarchy with a population of about 1.5 million Bahrainis and upwards of 600,000 migrant labourers from a number of different countries in the middle and Far East. Although a relatively small country, less than half the size of Ireland or Scotland, Bahrain's location at the heart of the Persian Gulf coupled with its regional and international links meant that it was potentially very vulnerable to pandemic spread of COVID-19.

Linked by the King Fahd causeway to Saudi Arabia, with whom the kingdom enjoys a close relationship, Bahrain is a Muslim country with a slightly larger section of Shi'ites compared to Sunnis. The ruling Khalifa family belongs to the minority Sunnis, something which can give rise to communal tensions. Devout Shi'ites regularly travel on pilgrimage to the holy sites in Iran; on their return they receive an affectionate welcome from family and friends, eager to share the aura of the recent trip in warm embraces.

With an economy based on oil refining together with

aluminium production the country enjoys a good standard of living with well-developed, freely available education and health services. Specialist medical education and research is particularly well-organised with strong links to the Royal College of Surgeons of Ireland which has invested heavily in local training facilities in Manama.

In the second week in February 2020, I was contacted by the private office of HRH Crown Prince Salman with a request to travel to Bahrain to advise him and his team about the country's response to the emerging threat from coronavirus. Having seen the Sky News interview on February 1st, Prince Salman, First Deputy Prime Minister and defence minister, was concerned about his country's preparedness to cope with the virus if and when it arrived in the region. He was determined to be ready.

Despite having already established a Corona Task Force on 3 February, two days after the broadcast, the Prince had decided that he would leave no stone unturned to protect the people for whom he was responsible. His request was that I should visit Bahrain and work closely with his team to identify any weaknesses in the Task Force plans and recommend action to ensure that they were robust and effective. As a result of this invitation I was to make two field visits to Bahrain, from 22-25 February and from 7-11 March and continued to advise and be part of Bahrain's COVID Task Force remotely via Skype once further travel became impossible.

Shoe-leather epidemiology in Bahrain
History teaches us that when it comes to public-health emergencies Geoffrey Rose's prerequisite for a clean mind and dirty hands is paramount. When it comes to dealing with a novel virus of unknown properties of infectivity, clinical impact, capacity for mutation and temporal and geographic behaviour, the precautionary principle tempered by pragmatic and political

considerations must be the starting point and sound intelligence the foundation. Down the centuries from William Henry Duncan and John Snow the messages are loud and clear: serendipity favours the prepared mind, plagiarism is not a crime in public health, independent voices are crucial, shoe-leather epidemiology, coalition building, resourcefulness and pragmatism, humanitarianism and enlightened self-interest together with communication and public mobilisation are the foundations. Combined with strong leadership and multi-disciplinary teamwork, they are the key to success. Almost without exception Bahrain had adopted these principles under Crown Prince Salman, a Cambridge University graduate with an MPhil in history and a well-developed understanding of the danger posed by epidemics and the need for pre-emptive action.

At the time of my first visit, on 22 February, there had been not yet been any cases in Bahrain, unlike the UK. But there was growing concern about the situation in nearby Iran and suspicion that the Iranian government was withholding data about the true facts on the ground there. A particular worry was the threat posed by an estimated 2-3,000 Bahraini Shi'ite pilgrims who were believed to be visiting the holy sites in Iran at that time. Their return via different intermediary routes would pose a real test of the arrangements for keeping the virus out of the country.

Having convened a National Taskforce to combat the Coronavirus on 3 February, the Crown Prince had also established a War Room in the Medical Institute under the direction of Lt-Colonel Dr Manaf Al Quatani. He was a senior infectious disease consultant at the military hospital and alumnus of the Royal College of Surgeons of Dublin. This Taskforce had daily meetings with Bahrain's Health Council and its chairman, a senior medical member of the Bahrain government, Lt-General Sheikh Mohamed bin Abdulla Al Khalifa. Alongside the Crown Prince, in his palace secretariat was Isa Al Hammadi, the impressive Bahraini senior civil servant in charge of public information.

A 26-person multi-disciplinary team including information analysts, epidemiologists, and public-health consultants had been drafted in to the War Room where an information platform was being put together that included the Johns Hopkins University global Coronavirus data streams together with live feeds from the hospitals and clinics and national public-health laboratory in Manama. From the start, the Taskforce had unfettered access, real-time, to the raw public-health data it needed to fight the pandemic. It was precisely the type of information that PHE refused to share with its local offices during Britain's lockdown period. Already in February, Bahrain's clinical facilities were being reconfigured to provide increased numbers of bio-secure beds and so make them capable of managing infectious patients suffering from the most serious form of symptoms.

Following my first visit and as a result of our close examination of the arrangements in place, these vital live information feeds would be expanded to even greater granular detail. The Bahraini Taskforce included continuous data feeds on: Corona PCR test capacity, logistic supply-chain information on enzymes, reagents and swabs, Personal Protective Equipment (PPE), together with reports on the numbers of tests carried out and their results. Even the dedicated national telephone number '444' for any suspected cases led to a direct feed into the War Room.

This impressive initial response created a coherent coordination hub and an excellent central support line against which to explore the system in place on the ground. Following my second visit at the beginning of March this would be extended to include daily reports from the prisons and isolation facilities on any relevant reported sickness.

Refreshingly, the Crown Prince urged me to leave no stone

unturned and to be as critical and as meticulous as was necessary. Thus, the approach I adopted was to walk systematically the passenger and personnel routes through the ports of entry: the airport, seaport and the causeway linking Bahrain to Saudi Arabia along which thousands of trucks and cars moved around the region every day. Each of the hospitals and clinics that were to be used for testing and isolating potential cases were inspected along with Bahrain's public-health laboratory. Key informants were interviewed and rigorously interrogated, drilling down and forensically exploring for potential weaknesses in the environmental, social and clinical biosecurity, possible points of vulnerability through which this simple but adaptable virus might gain entry. In short, I covered ever angle the way I would have done it if I had still been Regional Director of Public Health for North-West England and gone through the preparations in my region.

The Task Force had moved quickly to increase clinical capacity by freeing up hospital beds, mobilising community clinics for triaging and testing suspected cases and upgrading wards and clinical areas to be able to care safely for patients suffering from serious infectious disease potentially requiring ventilation.

Nevertheless one matter of concern was the movement and potential flow of both patients and staff between 'clean' and possibly contaminated areas of the hospitals. Carefully walking the corridors and tracing the routes of all those who might frequent these spaces led to the identification of vulnerable points in both clinical and staff areas with appropriate modification together with the rigorous prevention of staff mixing between 'clean' and dirty areas enforced via colour-coded uniforms.

The second field visit from 6 March included two further visits to the War Room, close examination of a new apartment block that had been requisitioned as a dedicated quarantine facility and of a 4,000 person newly constructed quarantine facility, with three bio-secure, discrete zones for triaging returning travellers from

Iran and elsewhere with high levels of Coronavirus, and the main national prison. Strengths and weaknesses of the plans and arrangements were identified and reported back in detail to the Task Force, the Bahrain Health Council and to the Crown Prince for prompt action.

But excellent public-health communication was the other side of the medical bulwark against the looming pandemic. The Task Force was going to need to inform Bahrain's millions of inhabitants in an equally coherent manner.

Particular attention was paid to developing a national communications strategy based on openness and transparency with the public, including very frequent press and media conferences with extended and open Question and Answer sessions staffed by senior members of the government and Task Force. It was important that there was constant and consistent communication from many channels and that it was not just limited to a handful of people making pronouncements.

Like Britain, Bahrain is host to people from different cultures and with different languages. Overlooking this fact would have left a door open for the pandemic. This also needed to be addressed and Isa al Hammadi, in charge of communications, came up with creative solutions. This included messaging the entire smart-phone owning population with details of advice, the segmentation of messaging to be appropriate to different communities and language groups using different modalities of communication. It also meant the early establishment of a team within the Task Force to identify and rebut 'Fake News' and rumours on social media.

These measures were to prove crucial in securing the co-operation of the diverse communities of the country, not least when it came to suspending religious pilgrimages and Friday prayers at mosques. An early decision resulting from my first field visit in the third week of February was to suspend the Formula 1 racing event due to take place in Manama from March 20. And to act urgently on other mass-participant events.

The evolving Bahrain response in February/March
Although the prompt action by the Crown Prince in convening a Coronavirus Task Force and opening a War Room, before there were any cases of infection in the country, had created a sound base of preparedness, essential adaptations followed even at that early stage. The key ingredient for Bahrain's success was openness to review and the realisation that outside scrutiny was not an imposition but an essential plank of preparedness. It enabled the country, unlike the UK, to turn in a response that would be among the best in the world and would subsequently be highly commended by the Director General of WHO.

As a result of this openness an early vulnerability was exposed and immediately rectified: the inadequate capacity for virus testing, including PCR machines, reagents, enzymes and swabs. Prompt action enabled more than adequate supplies to be secured well ahead of the time they were needed. So much so that extensive testing and tracing of cases became the foundation of effective control. Operational failure to do this at the same stage would underlie the UK failure to get to grips with the crisis.

Other weaknesses that were identified during my first visit and acted upon included:

* The need for a coherent, rigorously evidence-based (as opposed to wishful thinking) narrative to galvanise the joint working of many different agencies and to inform the strategy of public engagement and communications.
* Awareness of weak links in the chain of control of the virus through the many possible environmental, social and biological and clinical entry points into the country, safe flows of potential patients through the clinical system, together with

robust Standard Operating Procedures with clarity of roles and responsibilities in many frontlines. Examples included protocols for case definition, mask wearing and handling the dead.

* Specific groups and settings that might be vulnerable and pose a risk for onward transmission: air passengers, especially religious pilgrims and members of aircrews and merchant-fleets; truck, taxi and bus drivers; clinical and front line health service staff; migrant workers living in labour camps; sex workers; prison officers and prisoners; residents of psychiatric and other long-stay facilities.

* Collaboration with international partners to ensure that best practice was being followed, systematic logging of daily situation reports, experiences and actions to inform future learning.

A healthy population will suffer less from a pandemic. At this early stage of the looming crisis, we even had time to see to opportunities to boost and reinforce national-health promotion priorities in relation to healthy lifestyles, self-care and health inequalities that might build community resilience should the worst case scenario come to pass.

This was all in sharp contrast to the UK, where government attention would turn to this aspect only in July, after the lockdown and in desultory fashion. By this time, in the absence of an organisation such as PHE coordinating coherent pandemic communications, Britain had been so overrun with so many conflicting messages from ministers or the prime minister that health seemed just another initiative by the prime minister or an ambitious minister to throw a headline at the crisis Britain was in.

Another one of the issues that came to light during my first visit to Bahrain was the vulnerability posed by the contrasting conditions and behaviours of different social groups. The plush

VIP facilities available at port of entry on the causeway from Saudi Arabia into the country were in extreme contrast to those for ordinary travellers and in particular for truck drivers.

As the virus spread in the UK, the vulnerability arising from the environmental conditions of disadvantaged communities converged with that arising from the behaviours of the privileged and of devout faith communities in placing themselves and their intimates at risk. Also, action was being proposed to test regularly and improve the environmental and living conditions of many of the migrant workers, who at times make up almost 40 per cent of the people living in the kingdom, whose accommodation might make them vulnerable and provide a vehicle for community outbreaks.

This assessment and the prompt action that followed came just in time. On the 24 February, the last day of my first field trip, the first case of coronavirus infection was confirmed. The patient was a tour guide for religious pilgrimages to the holy sites in Iran and tested positive a week after his return (figure shows positive test result on PCR machine monitor). Normally a local school bus driver, the patient had already ferried pupils from three schools on his bus and the contact and testing began in earnest.

By the second field visit on 7 March, most of the recommendations made in February had been implemented and there had been no further cases. Not only had the Formula 1 Grand Prix been cancelled, but also other large social events, mass gatherings and religious pilgrimages, a pro-active approach having been taken by the Crown Prince and the Bahraini Health Council acting on the advice of the Task Force.

Contacts had been made with the Global International Severe Acute Respiratory and Emerging Infections Consortium (ISARIC), and the Bahrain team members had begun to collaborate on COVID intelligence and therapeutic research with 24 other countries.

Weekly screening of frontline health workers for Coronavirus was being put in place and extended to passengers and crew arriving at the international airport, where triage was now routine, backed up with systematic isolation of those who might be carrying the virus. Following a visit to the main prison, where over-crowding was identified as a risk, 901 prisoners were pardoned who were near the end of their sentences and who were believed to pose no risk to the community. A rapid-response team was being assembled to contact trace, isolate and treat those might become ill in localised outbreaks

Bahrain's comprehensive and pro-active instead of reactive approach would pay handsome dividends in limiting the health impact of the pandemic but also in shielding Bahrain's economy from the worst.

Bahrain, June 2020
The proof of the pudding is in the eating. In an international webinar hosted by the Bahraini Ambassador to the UK on 9 June 2020, Lt-Colonel Dr Al Quatani, the Taskforce's clinical lead, was able to report a success story for COVID-19, at least as far as the first wave was concerned.

In February and March field hospitals and quarantine facilities had been constructed, doubling the numbers of beds in the national healthcare system; Polymerase Chain Reaction (PCR) testing capacity had been increased from 800 to 8,800 tests per day, all arrivals at the airport were being tested, with reduced numbers owing to the suspension of admission to the country by non-nationals; self-isolation bracelets to track home quarantine cases and assist in contact tracing was in place; home working had been activated for 70% of employees; drive-through, and mobile testing was in place and a static testing centre created at the International Exhibition Centre; hotels had been designated as isolation and treatment centres; as in the UK volunteers had been mobilised to assist with the pandemic and they totalled a number of 40,000—also seen as an opportunity to build bridges between the Sunni and Shi'ite communities and to unite a common purpose; and the numbers of health workers had been increased. International collaboration with clinical and research colleagues around the world meant that from the lessons learned in China and the very first cases Bahrain had the benefit of the dynamic emerging knowledge of the most effective treatment protocols with demonstrable impact on clinical outcomes.

The reward for Bahrain's thorough planning was that only a partial lockdown had been necessary. Although places of mass gathering including schools and universities, museums, sightseeing places, cinemas, gyms and sit-down restaurants, had been closed, shops and markets remained open in a controlled fashion. Gatherings of more than five people were banned and, also well-ahead of the UK, people were required to wear masks in public. Of note in the challenges generated during the emergency in Bahrain had been a spike in the number of cases detected during the holy festival of Ramadan, characterised by close family gatherings, something that was to arise among other faith communities in which communal celebration featured.

By June 9 Bahrain had tested the equivalent of 224,000 out of each million population, one of the leaders in the world. 15,945 cases had been diagnosed, of whom 68% had already recovered and been discharged from hospital with 27 COVID-19 deaths, a death rate of 0.2%, making it one of the lowest reported. This figure was not just a measure of Bahrain's success but probably one of its most reliable statistics in view of the large numbers of tests carried out.

Bahrain had tested from February onwards just about anyone suspected of having COVID symptoms, as well as anyone tracked and traced from a positive result. This was in stark contrast to

Britain. Even the word 'testing' translated into something very different in Britain.

COVID testing in Britain's NHS hospitals had commenced at the same time as in Bahrain, but Britain's Chief Medical Officer Chris Whitty had defined COVID as having three exclusive symptoms—a sharp new cough, fever or shortness of breath. This was despite the fact that the World Health Organization had defined eight symptoms in early February. Britain would only add another two, arguably COVID's most distinctive ones, on 28 May, a month before national pandemic lockdown was to end: a loss of taste and smell.

Whitty's elliptical list of symptoms was not merely meant to inform Britain's physicians. It was prescriptive and there to control the levers of the colossal administrative processes within the whole of the NHS. Testing was permitted only for those patients who had the symptoms on the list. Those who, for example, had the two symptoms that were added months later would remain unidentified as carriers until late May. A patient might well be actually infected with coronavirus, but without the three symptoms Whitehall wasn't interested.

Britain's laboratories refused to accept testing requests from senior consultants in NHS hospitals for patients who didn't fit Whitehall's definition. When queried by Reuters' investigative reporters about this a PHE spokesperson said, 'That is right, but there is nothing unusual in this. Lab testing capacity was used to establish whether people that met the case-definition had the virus.' Further to Whitty's COVID definition, NHS physicians weren't so much testing for the presence of COVID in their patients as testing for its presence in a subset of carriers permitted by Whitehall, covering some but not all cases—up to only three fifths of infections based on the expanded list of approved symptoms. Senior doctors pleaded for the NHS's central COVID protocol to be amended to one that was realistic in their clinical experience. They had no success. While Westminster's medical diffidence may have had the result of saving some money on testing, it was also an easy way for the virus to ignore attempts to capture its carriers and for it to rapidly set up undetected bridgeheads within Britain, and to continue to do so for months.

In January other central restrictions on who could and could not be tested were imposed by geography on the NHS by Whitehall. At first it was restricted to only those linked to Wuhan who could be tested, then from 1 February it was the rest of China. Seven days later parts of Asia were added. Certain parts of Italy and Iran were included from February 25. But, before those dates, if an NHS doctor suspected that a patient with no ties to this growing succession of countries had COVID, centralised procedures would interfere with their attempt to test and find out.

Whitehall was the only one who could overrule the restrictions. Community testing organised by PHE followed similar limitations in testing and tracing outside hospitals. This didn't prevent minister for the cabinet office Michael Gove from having his daughter tested, sanctioned by Chief Medical Officer Chris Whitty.

Asked what he thought lay behind Bahrain's impressive performance Dr Al Quatani attributed it to three factors: testing, early treatment and communication. 'The major cause of death is late presentation, this is not a 'flu-like illness; come, we will test and treat you', he said. In contrast to the WHO view, and based on the trove of detailed, deep and rich data it has gathered, Bahrain's advice is that asymptomatic spread is a threat to the public, 'Our data showed 44% of those asymptomatic were infectious,' he said. 'We are small in size, but the power of the people of Bahrain is supporting each other to combat coronavirus'. An example of the ambition and pro-active interventions made during the emergency included the demolition of poor-quality housing estates for migrant labourers and their replacement with new building built to a high environmental health specification.

Early on in the pandemic, when news of Bahrain's achievements was mentioned, it was common to dismiss it as irrelevant to the UK as it was so different in size. It betrayed the closed-mindedness of Britain as opposed to the open approach in Bahrain. It also misunderstood that, as far as the pandemic was concerned, Westminster treated the rest of Britain as if it was the size as Bahrain and Whitehall as the sole pivot for a population of 70 million. Instead of dismissing solutions out of hand, Bahrain was ready to assess knowledge and expertise on its merits, that is whether it would strengthen the defences of its population against the pandemic. Even a cursory glance at Bahrain's over 40% migrant population would have made it clear how much there was to learn for a country such as Britain with fewer than 10% foreign-born inhabitants. Britain, however, looked stubbornly through the wrong side of the telescope.

As the emergency has unfolded, and with it the disaster of the centralised response by London and Whitehall, the clamour has grown louder for a much more local approach in which public-health teams can be fully engaged with the communities they know and understand.

One only has to point out that the Liverpool City Region is similar in population size to the Kingdom of Bahrain. By the beginning of June there had been over 500 deaths in Liverpool, equivalent to a mortality rate of almost five times higher than that of Bahrain. Then there are the economic consequences of a complete lockdown that are about to create havoc for a generation. None of this will be the case in Bahrain as a result of the first COVID wave.

What might it have been if, say, the Liverpool local director of Public Health had had the same authority and capacity to lead the COVID response from January as their Bahraini counterparts, rather than being controlled centrally from London, one-size fits all, like an oil tanker (but one with several captains at the helm pulling the rudder in different directions)?

As a regional director I have worked closely with many local Public Health Directors on fast-moving health emergencies. I know that they would have approached the as-yet unknown threat in exactly the same methodical way as the Bahrain government did. The advice the Crown Prince called me to Bahrain for, is precisely what would have been the standard part of my job. They would realise that data speed is of the essence and that, as a pandemic doesn't attack systemically but in specific locations, knowing where the virus is both crucial for fighting it and for not paralysing the area that is free from the virus.

There is a great similarity between public-health in moments of crisis and the military. The enemy doesn't attack everywhere at once. Like the military, local public-health officials are used to being both regimented and have great autonomy to make operational decisions on the battlefield. If General Patton would have had to wait for Winston Churchill's missives to reach him by way of General Eisenhower for every move, instead of receiving an objective, how could the Battle of Bulge not have become a never-ending disaster?

Like Patton, local Public Health Directors would give their right arm to fight street by street, corner by corner, like Wiltshire Public Health Director Daszkiewicz hunting down the nerve-agent, to prevent deaths and unnecessary mayhem, while informing the public on safety. As it was, they were tied behind their desks dealing with memoranda from their PHE bosses and with those from their local authority managers.

7

A Wasted Month
and an
Absentee Prime Minister

As the Coronavirus arrived in the UK prime minister Boris Johnson had a lot on his plate. He had recently left his second wife, Marina Wheeler, for another woman, Carrie Simmons, with the loose ends of another relationship still swirling around. He had won a general election, finally 'Got Brexit Done', and was about to become a father for a number of times that was publicly uncertain. Meanwhile he had managed to fit in an extended Christmas holiday to the private Caribbean island of Mustique. He was on this vacation when the first reports of the Coronavirus reached the World Health Organization on 31 December, and the newly re-elected prime minister was planning another break for February with his pregnant fiancée at the seventeenth-century grace-and-favour mansion of Chevening in Kent. Chequers, the sixteenth-century country house in Buckinghamshire usually reserved for the prime minister, was undergoing repair work. There he would be finalising the arrangements for his divorce from his estranged wife.

Problems started to pile up from the beginning of the year. Britain was hit by severe flooding, but there was to be no COBR meeting unlike during the flooding in November. Kent was one of the areas particularly hit, but Johnson made no visits to stricken areas as he had done while campaigning. His response to the rise of COVID showed the same pattern. Although this emergency ostensibly warranted a COBR meeting on 24 January, Johnson missed it, and according to a major investigative report in the *Sunday Times* on April 16, would go on to miss four more meetings before chairing his first on 2 March. Missing five of them was unprecedented behaviour for a prime minister when faced with a major national emergency.

With the exception of one typically superficial and self-aggrandising intervention in a speech at Greenwich on 3 February, and a flight of fancy on 11 February, about constructing a bridge between Northern Ireland and Scotland, something that was met with general ridicule, Boris Johnson was seemingly silent. His apparent concern at that point was that, as he stated on 3 February, 'there is a risk that new diseases such as coronaviruses will trigger a panic and a desire for market segmentation that go beyond the medically rational to the point of doing real and unnecessary economic damage.' Grandiloquently he also added, 'humanity needs some government somewhere that is willing at least to make the case powerfully for freedom'. The next months would make clear that as far as he, Dominic Cummings and his cabinet were concerned, humanity and the British people would have to look elsewhere rather than rely on him while his government stood in the way of the free exchange of public data on COVID inside and outside the government.

By February 9 the total number of reported infectious cases from China passed 40,000, with over 900 deaths. Also, 376 cases had been reported in other countries. On Monday February 10, the *Guardian* reported that the number of confirmed cases in the UK had doubled from four to eight. The previous week a Sussex businessman had been diagnosed as the third person having contracted the virus. He was one of 109 at a conference in

Singapore three weeks before—of which one attendee had come from Wuhan. He subsequently came to be implicated in the onward transmission to at least 11 Britons in three countries, acquiring the sobriquet of a 'superspreader'. From Singapore, Walsh had flown to his family staying at a ski-chalet near the Mont Blanc, France, with five later falling ill there. On his return within a week to Hove, Sussex, another four people on the chalet holiday tested positive in the UK, and a further member of the skiing party fell ill returning to Mallorca. In Britain, the cases with links to Mr Walsh included two doctors at a surgery in Brighton, which had to suspend seeing its patients in order not to spread the disease. The connection with ski resorts as bridgeheads of forward transmission was soon to snowball in the UK and elsewhere.

The following day it was reported that a student at the University of Sussex was being tested for the virus, arousing close to a panic on the campus, although his test result was subsequently reported negative. and the numbers of those in quarantine at Arrowe Park reached 100 as more travellers arrived back from Wuhan. The same day the Coronavirus was given its official name of COVID-19 by Dr Tedros of WHO, who told a press conference that a name was decided that 'did not refer to a geographical location, an animal, an individual or a group of people, and which is also pronounceable and related to the disease... having a name matters to prevent the use of other names that can be inaccurate or stigmatising'. While the Director General of WHO was establishing himself as the global face and voice of trust for the emerging pandemic, the same could not be said for his opposite numbers in the UK.

Faced with a pandemic public-health emergency it is essential to have clear and accurate communications at both national and local levels, delivered consistently by figures who come to be recognising as worthy of trust and respect. In this respect the British government got off to a poor start as a result of a vendetta that had begun in December 2019 when Boris Johnson lay siege to the BBC with a two-pronged attack. Accusing the Corporation of anti-Tory bias, he threatened to decriminalise non-payment of the license fee and, in addition, he had imposed a boycott for ministers on the Today Programme, with its long history of setting the daily political agenda of the country. Not only had the prime minister disappeared stage left to Chevening, he had also sabotaged two of the main communication channels through which information about the looming pandemic would have to be distributed.

As he was no longer present, there was furthermore confusion who was the political face of the emergency. Bizarrely, this vacuum was something that was to continue in the weeks and months ahead, with a succession of walk-on roles for ministers and their deputies of all plumage, none of whom had the prime-minister's power to make decisions. From the point of view of an authoritative voice for public health this was nothing short of disastrous.

Meanwhile, the newly appointed Chief Medical Officer, Chris Whitty was being kept back. Eventually, with rising concern as to how this was playing with the public, the government broke its own embargo and let Professor Whitty out to appear on the Today Programme at 8.15am on Thursday 13 February.

The Chief Medical Officer took the opportunity of introducing his proposed framework for dealing with the virus in the UK, consisting of four strands—'contain, delay, mitigate, research'. This dry approach gave no hint as to what practical measures were to be followed but was nevertheless to assume the status of a mantra over the next few weeks, taking its place alongside the governments reassuring claims to be 'following the science'.

As the emergency unfolded Professor Whitty would struggle to establish himself as an authoritative voice. New in the job, he both struggled to rise to the occasion and with the fact that the government was already on the backfoot, lagging the news cycle.

It was even worse. In the absence of the head of government making decisions, the Chief Medical Officer and the Chief Scientific Adviser were advanced by cabinet ministers as their praetorian guard who would deflect any adverse future criticism and jeopardy to their ministerial positions.

Chris Whitty's background was primarily that of a clinician and academic epidemiologist. He had little traditional frontline public-health experience and appeared to have a lack of assertiveness with the politicians. Despite his congenial presence and initial credibility, he would, rightly or wrongly, increasingly come to be seen as the fall guy for government as it sought to deflect blame for slow and wrong decisions taken by the cabinet. Whitty would finally find his voice in July, by which time the cosy relationship between the politicians and their advisers had begun to break down

Where Bahrain was by now establishing control over movement of large groups of people in and out of the kingdom in preparation of the pandemic, the Johnson government, with no one in charge, slid absent-mindedly towards the half-term exodus of British families. Parliament went into recess on Thursday 13 February and the schools broke up for the holidays the following day with thousands of families migrating off to the ski slopes abroad or to their second homes in scenic areas around Britain such as the lakes in South Cumbria.

The infection-spree in the first week of February connected to Brighton businessman Steve Walsh at a French ski resort was a portent of things to come. During the first half of February, cases of COVID virus had begun to occur in the ski-resort areas of northern Italy and Austria where the spread of the virus had acquired an accelerating momentum. Later analysis of previously taken samples of sewage water would indicate that the virus had been circulating in Italy from as early as December 2019. This tallied with satellite evidence that China had under-reported the beginning of COVID-19. By February 21 Italy was reporting 51 cases of infection and two deaths and by 29 this had risen exponentially to 1,128 cases and 21 deaths. British families were by now vacationing in these areas.

With the virus circulating freely in the mountain-resort areas, it is highly likely that families returning from these ski slopes will have been carriers, seeding outbreaks in their own communities at the end of their holiday break. If this was indeed the case those infected would have themselves become unwell and infectious around the turn of the month. They would begin to appear in the hospital admission statistics and deaths by the third week in March. By this time both diagnosed cases and deaths in the UK were doubling every 2-3 days, reaching 1140 confirmed cases and 21 deaths by 14 March.

As the numbers of cases in the UK began to creep up during February, Public Health England (PHE) had initiated the process of testing those who might be ill with the virus and tracing their immediate contacts. PHE's local Directors of Public Health were charged with executing this and instructed to send the tests back to the central Colindale laboratory. The numbers of cases during this 'Slow Burn' phase of the outbreak remained relatively small but the local directors were not given the results which people tested positive.

The problem would come when the epidemic curve moved on to become a 'Rising Tide'. It would require exponential testing capacity within the community. Until the formation of PHE in 2013, local Public Health Directors would have assessed testing capacity in their area and decided themselves where to send the test in order to get the most urgent response. Instead, tests started piling up at Colindale, while the laboratory got further and further behind. Within a month the system would run out of capacity and community testing would stop.

While the virus was making its way into the nooks and crannies of the vulnerable and elderly via bridgeheads formed by their relatives returning from half-term holidays abroad, the epidemiological advisers to government were beginning to test their models of epidemic spread.

On 20 February the government issued an update of its 'Guidance for Pandemic 'flu' that had previously been updated on 24 November 2017. At this stage, working off historic influenza planning assumptions, the guidance was postulated that around 50% of the population might become infected and that the UK could experience up to 750,000 additional deaths over the course of a pandemic.

According to the epidemiologists, 'these figures might be expected to be reduced by the impact of countermeasures, but the impact of such mitigation is not certain. The combination of particularly high-attack rates and severe disease, resulting in this deaths figure, is also relatively (but unquantifiably) improbable. Taking account of this, and the practicality of different levels of response, when planning for excess deaths, local planners have been set the target of preparing... up to 210,000 to 315,000 additional deaths, (representing a 1% mortality rate), possibly over as little as a 15-week period and perhaps half of those over 3 weeks at the height of the outbreak.'

It was an arresting but curious guidance. It assumed that there was neither prevention nor containment other than hand washing and personal hygiene by the British population. The epidemiologists made no reference to lessons learned from the SARS pandemic of 2002-3. Nor was there any mention of the role of local Directors of Public Health in stemming the pandemic. While no doubt academically fascinating, it wasn't an accurate reflection of reality on the ground. The Bahrain Task Force would have sent it back for redrafting.

As the first UK case of person-to-person transmission was reported on 29 February there was the sense of an absentee prime minister leading a four-day-a-week government was cementing itself. Johnson was not the only one. That PHE, the agency based in London responsible for overseeing the protection of the nation's health, seemed not to work weekends would become apparent in the weeks to come. Already late in responding, it depended on what day of the week it was whether something might be done or not. It led to fits and starts and 'doing too much too late'.

Meanwhile other countries where the virus had been first to arrive, including mainland China and its near-neighbours Hong Kong, Taiwan, South Korea and Thailand were taking vigorous action. Responding promptly to any outbreaks, they tested, traced and isolated those affected. But these countries also embraced a wide range of social and environmental measures, quarantining or locking down whole communities, street disinfecting, mandating home working, banning mass events, encouraging social distancing, enforcing the wearing of masks, and instigating school closures where there were outbreaks. By this time I was in Bahrain and followed these developments closely with the Task Force, and in our discussions we fine-tuned their on-going preparations for when the virus would strike in the country.

With anxiety growing and the virus accelerating around the world, pressure was growing on WHO to declare a pandemic. I had the good fortune of being in Bahrain with unencumbered access to all the relevant facts, much in the way as I would have been as a UK Regional Director of Public Health in the first decade of the century. It certainly looked like a pandemic as viewed from the War Room in Bahrain, with its Johns Hopkins University live feed of global COVID cases.

With the accelerating deterioration in Italy and in close proximity to Iran, where under-reporting was highly likely amid reports of increasing chaos, this moment seemed to have already arrived. Interviewed from Manama on 24 February on Channel 4

News by Cathy Newman, I took the opportunity to press for urgent action in Britain, too, asserting that 'to all intents and purposes this is a pandemic... It requires the organised efforts of everybody'.

It would take the Director General of WHO another two weeks to declare COVID a global pandemic. Bahrain was in excellent shape for the battle ahead. Britain was in no recognisable shape.

8

A Floating Petri Dish

Maggi Morris

Meanwhile there was one news story that transfixed the global media. It was one that should have given even a myopic politician pause for thought.

The Diamond Princess cruise ship, carrying 2,666 passengers and 1,045 crew from 56 different countries, left the port of Yokohama in Tokyo Bay, Japan, on 20 January 2020. It was outward bound on a Lunar New Year's voyage of Southeast Asia. Full of anticipation, guests were looking forward to a leisure packed cruise of fine dining, 'bottomless buffets', endless entertainment and celebration of anniversaries, drinking from champagne fountains, and bathing in tranquil Japanese Olsen pools. Little did they realise that they were about to find themselves at an epicentre of the COVID-19 pandemic. One month later, on February 20, it was confirmed that the ship had more cases of the new Coronavirus than anywhere else outside China.

In any epidemic, one of the priorities for public-health teams is to identify the first or index case and track and trace outwards to contain the outbreak. In the case of the Diamond Princess the search led to an 80-year-old resident of Hong Kong who had briefly visited Shenzhen, in the Guangdong province of mainland China for just a few hours on January 10 before returning home to Hong Kong.

On January 17, he travelled to Tokyo where two days later he developed a cough before boarding the ship the following day in Yokohama to travel home. Having disembarked on January 25 in Hong Kong he developed a fever on January 30, and on February 1 the Hong Kong public-health authorities announced their first case—an 80-year-old male patient. It seems likely that from the point of view of subsequent events on the ship this man was the index case, although whether there was already somebody else incubating the virus on board is unknown.

Returning from Hong Kong to Yokohama, the Diamond Princess put in to the port of Okinawa, where most of the passengers went ashore. None were reporting symptoms of coronavirus infection. The ship continued its return to Yokohama where the captain, Genaro Arma, docked early at the request of the Japanese authorities. It did so on 3 February at Daikoku pier, a massive container warehouse island. Although further excursions ashore were cancelled, at that point social mixing and entertainment on the ship continued. But already passengers and crew were beginning to manifest early symptoms of infection and soon the vessel was to be plunged into quarantine under the Japan's quarantine laws.

On February 5 testing began for those exhibiting symptoms. It was rapidly extended to the elderly and others regarded as being at high risk, the average age of passengers being 70 years. Initially the Japanese authorities made the erroneous assumption that there was no spread of infection on board the ship. It allowed those who were asymptomatic or testing negative to disembark, a decision that was subsequently severely criticised.

The Diamond Princess was by now a floating Petri dish, incubating the virus among all those living in close quarters, in cabins and below decks. Had everybody been disembarked, tested, triaged and isolated at this time further transmission may have been avoided and lives saved.

Following confirmation of the first 10 cases among those still onboard and recognising the possibility of community person-to-person transmission, the Japanese ministry of health instigated a 14-day quarantine and observation period. On day 5 of the quarantine a decision was taken to move to mass testing at the end of the 14 days. Fatefully, no mention was made of testing the crew.

The Japanese response to the outbreak on the Diamond princess was widely criticised as *ad hoc*, lax and chaotic, and it changed its approach on February 13th, day 9 of the quarantine, allowing the disembarkation first of the elderly and later of others who were testing COVID negative. Controversially the British passengers together with the crew, were among the last to leave the vessel.

In retrospect it seems that there was little preparedness for managing an outbreak such as that caused by COVID-19 and that the response to the situation aboard the Diamond Princess, as with other cruise liners during the pandemic, was sub-standard. Clues as to the potential for viral spread on board ships are to be found both generally in the history of navigation. and more specifically in the pandemic of influenza in 1918-19, when infection onboard military vessels on the eastern seaboard of the US was incriminated in the spread of the virus between military bases.

In recent years, outbreaks of winter vomiting caused by the small round virus (norovirus) have been quite common on board cruise ships. This virus can be quite readily transmitted on door fixtures, handrails and bathroom fittings. The rapid growth of the leisure-cruise market over the past ten years should have prompted a review of public-health and safety measures. But none of the governments involved had undertaken such a review of this booming area of the global economy.

There can be little doubt that comprehensive testing for COVID should have been conducted on all passengers and crew from the moment the first cases appeared. That this didn't happen appears to have been both on account of the costs to the private sector and the shortage of testing capacity among the public authorities.

The decision to dock the vessel in Okinawa with potentially infected passengers mixing onshore may have contributed to spread among both passengers and among the community where there was mixing. But the decision to keep most people on board, converting the ship into what was essentially a floating Petri dish was the most contentious decision. In the event 3,711 people underwent a 14 day quarantine aboard the vessel, over 700 tested positive for the virus and 9 died. It is estimated that at least one third of those on board were infected with the virus by the end of the episode but that many were asymptomatic. The rapid spread of the virus over a short number of days suggests that a large number of the latter were infectious, despite being asymptomatic. The Bahraini Task Force had calculated 44% after analysis of its data, but this conclusion is still contested by WHO.

While placing the ship in quarantine may have reduced transmission among the passengers, but not among the crew, immediate evacuation of all passengers and crew with onshore isolation may have reduced the toll. A relatively manageable burden of care from a light seasonal 'flu impact in 2019-2020 meant that Japan would have been well positioned with clinical capacity to provide adequate care for passengers and crew onshore.

For those who were paying attention, the Diamond Princess was a microcosm of the issues that would soon come to be projected on the national canvas. Attention to the quality of life aboard ship in the extreme circumstances of such quarantine, as experienced by those on board the Diamond Princess, goes beyond the minimum necessary to survive. Shortages of medicines were being reported as early as day 2. Despite special efforts for those with illnesses such as diabetes and heart disease shortages remained.

Unable to be repatriated people felt trapped on board.

Passengers and crew soon experienced mental stress. Mental-health support should be part of emergency planning for cruise ships.

This is not to say that spontaneous help was not forthcoming from civic society. Local school children sent a video message to all on board saying 'We Are With You' and a banner from the people 'Yokohama Stands by You' was displayed around the pier. On day 11, February 15, a private tech company helped with a request from the Japanese ministry of health to provide 2,000 iPhones for passengers to send requests for medications and receive free health consultations. A disaster psychiatric-assistance team was despatched to the scene but it seems that concerns about infection control impeded its intervention.

The events on the Diamond Princess illustrated two different approaches to the spread of a contagious disease, isolation and quarantine. Although conceptually clear, they are complex in practise due to legal and social issues as well as the practicalities of an emergency situation.

Isolation is the term used for those who are confirmed to be infected with a communicable disease and are being kept isolated from the healthy population. In contrast the term quarantine is used to describe the separation and restriction of movement of those who have been exposed to infection to see if they become sick. People who are quarantined may have been exposed but may or may not know whether this is indeed the case.

There is a dilemma between enforced quarantine of those who may or may not pose a hazard to others and the isolation of those who most likely do. The issues raised of individual (human) rights versus their responsibilities to the group and the group's interests are fundamental ones which are at the heart of many public-health questions. They have been writ large not only with regard to quarantine and isolation but also the broader question of lockdown as a strategy for containment of the pandemic.

The deployment of isolation, quarantine and lockdown, are interventions that follow a classical public-health strategy. They are connected with the nineteenth-century utilitarian moral philosophy of 'the greatest good of the greatest number', as proposed by British philosophers Jeremy Bentham and the more nuanced John Stuart Mill, who wrote 'freedom only deserves that name as long as it doesn't deprive others of theirs'. In the US it is pithily translated to the twenty-first century as, 'your freedom ends where my nose begins'.

Applied to the Diamond Princess in February 2020, these measures not only turned dream holidays sour for passengers but also turned the jobs of the crew into a nightmare. The baseline for intervention in either case was very different, the lower one creating a fertile breeding ground for the virus.

The 1,045 strong crew was mainly drawn from low- and middle-income countries in South East Asia in contrast to the passengers who were from high-income countries. The crew lived in multi-bunked accommodation in the bowels of the ship whilst the passengers were for the most part in cabins with windows, perhaps with balconies although some were in windowless, interior cabins.

While many of the passengers were vulnerable to infection with COVID by virtue of their age and pre-existing health conditions, the younger crew were potentially at risk because of their close proximity to others in cramped accommodation. Furthermore, the nature of the crews' responsibilities meant that they were moving freely between areas of the ship where infection might be contracted. In addition to their regular duties for provision of general services and potentially contaminated laundry, of necessity the crew also became the care givers to the passengers.

A major issue raised by the Diamond Princess as a quarantine vessel is the extent to which this exacerbated or contained the ship-borne outbreak. Whilst the alternative of disembarking everybody at the outset and triaging them into some alternatives of fit-for-purpose isolation and quarantine onshore might have prevented the extensive spread that occurred on board, once passengers were confined to their cabins the spread of symptomatic patients declined. Although cabin quarantine seems to have reduced further spread there were reports of the measure being loosely applied with some passengers breaking the one-hour-a-day of freedom for those with no-cabin windows (alternate days for others).

As for the crew, their situation was not so fortunate and the spread of infection continued among them well after February 5.

It has been suggested that in the constrained crew accommodation the air ventilation may have facilitated person to person spread, a precursor of discussions about the safety of office spaces much later.

The Diamond Princess episode was also an early test case for other closed communities on shore, with lessons for epidemic spread in care homes and prisons. The importance of transmission in communal areas such as gyms, cinemas and dining rooms is where much of the early infection will have occurred. A second wave of infection among crew members, following the first wave among passengers, demonstrates the crucial importance of a nuanced multi-disciplinary approach to environmental and social, non-medical interventions and subtly different vectors between social groups, to prevent secondary spread.

The most deafening warning sign was, however, that the Diamond Princess showed early on the initial vulnerability of an older population, many of whom would have underlying, predisposing health conditions. In Britain, judging by its lack of action, the Johnson cabinet seem to have ignored the tragedy's predictive value and dismissed it as—'nothing to do with us'.

9

Where There is No Vision, the People Perish

Proverbs 29:18

As February became March the epidemic was progressing relentlessly around the world. On March 1, CNN reported that the coronavirus had now killed more than 3,000 people worldwide, with the vast majority being in mainland China. There had been more than 88,000 cases globally with infections on every continent except Antarctica and the first cases had occurred in New York and California. 54 deaths had been reported from Iran, although the real tally was probably much higher, 34 from Italy and accelerating fast, 20 from Korea, 12 from Japan and one death each in the Philippines, Taiwan, Australia, Thailand and the US.

The first reported death in the UK was on 5 March, of a woman in her 70's living in a care home in Berkshire with another death, also that of a woman, at the Pennine acute hospital in Oldham, the same day. It subsequently transpired that the first three deaths had actually occurred two days earlier, on 3 March, in Nottingham, Essex and Buckinghamshire. Worryingly, there was no immediately obvious connection to these cases.

As other cases started piling up, the clinical characteristics of the as-yet unknown virus finally started to reveal themselves in the first victims of the pandemic. With a timeline of between 5-14 days incubation period, cases that were potentially linked to the half-term skiers presented symptoms of clinical infection. At first these symptoms were reported to be not dissimilar to those of 'flu with a sore throat, high temperature and a new, continuous cough. Later it would be realised that a far wider range of symptoms could also occur, including headache, sometimes gastrointestinal symptoms, and also particularly the sudden loss of taste and smell.

Ominously, evidence began to accumulate that some infected people could be contagious before they manifested any symptoms and that many people could experience infection and recover from it without feeling significantly poorly. Meanwhile, they might have been contagious. Children, in particular, seemed less susceptible to infection with the severity increasing with each decade of life and especially poor outcomes among the over 60's and the very elderly.

As knowledge grew about the clinical illness caused by the virus, another pattern emerged in which after between about 7-10 days patients either recovered or became significantly worse. A worsening clinical picture was characterised by Acute Respiratory Distress (ARD), requiring hospitalisation and, potentially, artificial ventilation. In turn this could be followed by a catastrophic immune-system over-response known as a cytokinetic storm in which multiple organs could experience extensive damage associated with inflammatory and thrombotic phenomena. Among these patients the course of the illness tended to become critical towards the end of the third week when recovery or death followed a clinical crisis.

Taken together, these components of the clinical epidemic would point towards patients who had contracted their illness on the half-term ski slopes becoming unwell towards the end of February with a proportion requiring hospitalisation during the first week or so. They would be impacting on the numbers of deaths around the middle of the March.

Although globally the numbers of cases and affected countries continued to accelerate, the WHO was still reluctant to call the pandemic. The implication of such a move is administrative, but the move has enormous symbolic value. In the past WHO was criticised when a pandemic turned out to be less threatening than anticipated. 'Pandemic' status carried the potential for galvanising international health diplomacy in both a good and a potentially negative way for the organisation.

Finally, having missed the first five meetings of COBR on COVID, Prime Minister Johnson attended and chaired his first meeting on Monday 2 March. The virus was already rampant through the country. The following day he appeared on television from 10 Downing Street, flanked by the Chief Medical Officer, Professor Chris Whitty and the government's Chief Scientific Adviser, Sir Patrick Vallance, with two union flags. You didn't need to recall Johnson's previous public address, by now a month ago, during which he had spent florid verbiage on superman's flowing cape, or x-ray vision to see through the strained symbolism.

At this, the first of what were to become almost daily press conferences, Boris Johnson launched his Coronavirus Action Plan. Essentially, it was a repeat of Whitty's four strands of 'contain, delay, research and mitigate'. Inexplicably, he went on to say that 'for the overwhelming majority of people who contract the virus, this will be a mild disease from which they will speedily and fully recover.' There was no clinical proof of this as yet whatsoever.

There was no plan either, just statements pinned to qualifiers such as 'fabulous' and 'well-prepared'. 'Let's not forget', the prime minister said, 'we already have a fantastic NHS, fantastic testing systems and fantastic surveillance of the spread of disease… Our country remains extremely well-prepared, as it has been since the outbreak began in Wuhan, several months ago'.

Almost as a throw-away line, Johnson added, 'crucially we must not forget what we can all do to fight this virus, which is to wash our hands… with soap and water… wash your hands with soap and hot water for the length of time it takes to sing Happy Birthday twice'. It was a leaf from the same sloppy and imprecise script (which one was it, was it 'water' or 'hot water' that would prevent COVID transmission according to the prime minister?) as PHE's unreliable *novichok* laundry advice in 2018 to the inhabitants of Salisbury.

As Johnson spoke, the so-called 'containment' phase of 'his' plan was already failing. Testing, tracing and isolating would be abandoned in some ten days largely as a result of the Colindale pile-up. Systemic lockdown of the country, which would pummel the British economy was only three weeks away.

Well-prepared, Bahrain was able to avoid this measure and Johnson's speech compared poorly to the business-like visit I had with Bahrain's Crown Prince to the Task Force on 23 February, the day before I left. He identified the problems that lay ahead, identified a clear objective (a low infection rate) and that Bahrain's 'public-health-prevention measures to keep abreast with international developments' would be the priority. It should have been the model for the prime minister's rambling speech and dubious information on COVID.

More chaos followed in the government's messaging. Two days later, as some of his advisers were recommending the abandonment of hand-shakes and hugs, the prime minister was continuing to shake hands and went on the record as saying that he had visited a hospital 'where I think there were coronavirus patients and I was shaking hands with everybody, you will be pleased to know, and I continue to shake hands'. How Boris Johnson knew that his behaviour would not lead to virus-transmission was not clear. Had he read his COBR briefings without his Clark Kent glasses (or visited Krypton)?

The front page of the *Sunday Times* on 8 March led with a story that Whitehall was planning for the worst as the virus spread. Reporting that Boris Johnson would be chairing only his second COBR meeting the following day the newspaper wrote that medical experts were expected to move formally into the Whitty's second, 'delay', phase of the government's response and that this could lead to more people working from home and fewer public gatherings. What was media speculation in Britain were measures that had been widely implemented elsewhere since February. Officials in Whitehall were describing a 100,000 figure as the central estimate for the number of deaths from the virus, as opposed to the earlier worst case scenario of 500,000 deaths if 80% of the population was affected. Whitehall had not released the latter figure in order to avoid wide-spread panic.

While the tight circle of yea-sayers around Johnson pretended there was nothing to see, exam boards were drawing up plans to delay GCSE and A-level exams. It was the beginning of another Westminster cyclone that would hit, on this occasion, Britain's teenagers and their future. Here, too, the Johnson cabinet would in the end exacerbate rather than mitigate the knock-on effect of their pandemic measures. The chancellor of the exchequer was planning a budget to 'turn on the spending taps if the crisis prompts a recession' and Lindsay Hoyle, the Speaker of the House of Commons was rumoured to be planning a ban on visitors to the House and to favour closing parliament for three months.

The other lead story was that, after a grim day in which the number of known cases had jumped from 1,200 to 5,833 with 200 deaths so far, the Italian government was proposing to seal off a large swathe of the north of the country to stem the spread of the coronavirus, that all ski resorts would be closed and weddings and funerals cancelled. While Bahrain had already cancelled mass events, the culture secretary was to hold meetings on the Monday to decide whether to abandon sporting events or to hold them behind closed doors.

Meanwhile in the UK newspapers, the inside pages carried a glowing photograph of the prime minister with his new fiancée and her £10,000 emerald engagement ring enjoying the England against Wales rugby match at Twickenham, which England won

33-30; and most of page 4 was taken up with a report of Meghan Markle's last appearance as the Duchess of Sussex before moving to North America, visiting a comprehensive school in Dagenham.

Towards the centre pages there were details on how the 'contain, delay, mitigate' parts of the Johnson-Whitty plan were intended to be executed. It included the early release of prisoners and the possible scrapping of refuse collections whilst raising concerns over the prospect of hospital patients spilling into corridors. Attention was also given to the arrival back home two weeks ago of 39 passengers who had been on board the cruise liner Grand Princess at the same time as a man who died in a hospital in California diagnosed with COVID. They had been sent an email from its cruise operator Carnival saying, 'If you have experienced any symptoms of acute respiratory illness with fever, chills or cough since your return home, please immediately contact your medical provider'. PHE declined to say whether the 39 travellers had been contact-traced. Why? Presumably because the answer was no and the organisation didn't want to admit it had not stuck to the plan.

By Monday 9 March 319 cases had been confirmed in the UK nationally together with the 5th death. In the press conference that followed a meeting of COBR, Boris Johnson was again not on top of his brief and reported it as the fourth. He went on to say that, looking around the world, containment was unlikely to work on its own. He might instead have trained his mind on the country he was in charge of. Whereas there was a reluctance to learn from other countries, particularly close neighbours in Europe, what was happening elsewhere in 'the world' would become another often-heard phrase whenever the government announced that plans failed to yield results.

As his government was lurching to the 'delay' phase, Johnson sought to reassure the public that 'we are doing everything we can to combat this outbreak, based on the very latest scientific and medical advice'. He repeated that 'the best thing we can all do is wash our hands for 20 seconds in soap and water'. It was to be a much-repeated mantra, even though the transmission profile of the virus was as yet a mystery to doctors and clinical scientists. Infections on the Princess Diamond already presented the question to scientists whether viral infections might be caused by aerosols. Anything called the 'latest' in the context of COVID meant by extension practically nothing at all for certain at this stage of the pandemic. Washing hands (but what about the population under the age of ten?) was a start but not the panacea the Johnson cabinet pretended it was in the absence of evidence.

Bahrain was very fortunate indeed to have the King and Crown Prince in charge instead. All the areas and regions, Bahrain sized or not, that constituted the geographical parts of in England Wales were not so lucky. They had the bad fortune of no longer having the autonomous public-health professionals they had had since William Duncan was first appointed as Medical Officer of Health by the City of Liverpool in 1837. Not only that, their local response teams were anchored to Boris Johnson and his cabinet, health minister Hancock's PHE, and treacly Whitehall.

Bahrain was, however, once like Liverpool—which is similar in population size. From 1892 to 1971, the country fell under London's rule as a protectorate and would have had to follow Whitehall's guidance to the letter. Had that still been the case in 2020, its population would have remained as unprotected as Britain's regions and cities were as a result of Westminster having taken away the power of local public-health officials to respond to the crisis without having to wait for the memo from Whitehall. London jealously clung, and continued to cling, to its central power even by August in the teeth of the evidence that its approach to what was happening in England and Wales had led to the least effective COVID handling in the world. What a difference it would have made on the impact of COVID and the economy if all the regions in Britain could have taken the initiative in the first week of February, like Bahrain did, even as London remained inert for inchoate political reasons.

10

SAGE

By Wednesday 11 March the tally had reached 596 cases and 10 deaths. The numbers were doubling exponentially every two to three days. But worse was to come and the country's public-health system was straining to keep up with the need to test and trace new cases, never mind isolate all those detected.

On January 30 the WHO had declared the spread of COVID as a Public Health Emergency of International Concern (PHEIC). Such a declaration is not necessarily confined to infectious disease and may cover an emergency caused by a chemical agent or radioactivity. The spread of COVID warranted it. Such declarations are defined as 'constituting an extraordinary event which is determined to constitute a public-health risk to other States through the international spread of disease and to potentially require a coordinated international response'.

Under the 2005 International Health Regulations the declaration of a PHEIC by an International Health Committee of experts required immediate international action; the mechanism was developed after the SARS pandemic of 2002. Although they are intended to have the force of law, their enforcement in practise is another matter.

Contrary to popular misconception, the World Health Organization is not a supranational body but an association of countries. It must work to achieve concerted action by member states through consensus and through diplomacy. In that sense a PHEIC is more of a 'call to action' than an instruction to its member states who are funding the organisation. Thus, policy choices for international outbreak management and control are not only fraught with attendant scientific uncertainty about the new threat. They are also wrapped up in political risk and subject to distortion by the potential for recrimination by aggrieved member nations and stakeholders.

Biting post-mortem criticism comes with the territory. Since 2009 there have been six PHEIC declarations, including the 2009 Swine 'flu pandemic, the 2014 Ebola epidemic and the COVID-19 outbreak. When the 2009 epidemic tailed off eighteen months later, leaving a tally of 17,000 deaths worldwide, the WHO was widely criticised. It was claimed the organisation had exaggerated the danger, influenced by the pharmaceutical industry with a special interest in selling anti-viral agents. In 2014, with the highly contagious and fatal Ebola virus in West Africa, WHO was again criticised. This time for being too slow to act.

Against this background, when Dr Tedros declared the Global Public Health Emergency for COVID-19 in January 2020, it should have been taken as the first shot across the bow that a pathogen attack was imminent. Most governments and their health professionals understood that it was time to start paying attention, as did, for example, Bahrain. Whitehall in the UK was an exception, choosing to downplay the PHEIC. It was not the first time. A sluggish response between the PHEIC and the WHO's global-pandemic warning was also a feature of Swine 'flu in 2009. When the pandemic fizzled out this gamble paid off. In reality, it is the PHEIC which should be seen as the trigger for national action and it is not easy to understand why Whitehall was the outlier among the WHO's member states.

From 1999 WHO has ascribed six phases to an emerging

epidemic in order to prime national preparedness and response planning and in order to allow its member states to walk the tight rope of an effective response that is a warranted addition to local public-health budgets. The guidance from WHO makes clear that these phases are not designed to predict what will happen during a pandemic, or that they will progress in sequence. It is merely a taxonomy of the threat.

The WHO's phases classify the spread of infection from phase one in which no viruses among animals have been reported to cause infections in humans, through phases two and three in which sporadic cases have occurred in humans without human-to-human spread, and on to phases four, five and six with progressive human-to-human spread, initially locally, and then progressively to at least two countries in one WHO region and finally to community-level spread in at least one country in more than one WHO region.

The WHO uses this schema as the basis of its declaration of a global pandemic. But it remains a judgement call based on many other things apart from the science. The upshot of all these disparate factors was that Dr Tedros moved on 11 March to declare the global pandemic of COVID.

Arriving back into Heathrow from my second field visit to Bahrain at 8 am on 11 March, and catching the shuttle up to Manchester airport, I was met by news that mental-health minister Nadine Dorries had tested positive with the virus after having been in No 10 Downing Street with the prime minister and she was now in isolation. The news also reported that a Vietnamese socialite had infected seven Brits who had shared a flight with her as she returned home from fashion shows in Paris and Milan.

The front-page of one broadsheet was, nonetheless, dominated by Boris Johnson and Carrie Symond's new dog. The top-of-the-line piece was complete with a staged, full-colour photo of 'Dillon', their Jack Russell cross. The chancellor, Rishi Sunak, was furthermore planning to fill 50 million potholes in roads. Redolent of John Major's 'cones line', it was part of Sunak's grand capital investment plan to level up the country of the type spoofed by The Thick of It's ministers with ambitions.

The COVID-19 news from Italy had gone from bad to worse. The number of recorded cases had risen from 10,149 to 12,462 in one day and the number of deaths from 631 to 827. With the north of the country now locked down, 20,000 British tourists were faced with the prospect of making their way home overland by the best means they could. A 60-year-old man from Manchester, who had already made it back from Italy, was the third person to die in Britain, with his family having to self-isolate and unable to say 'goodbye'. It was a bitter foretaste of many such family tragedies to come in Britain. A Liverpool surgeon who had recently returned from skiing in northern Italy and been working as usual was reported to have treated 50 patients before testing positive for the virus.

One in 20 cases was now being contracted within the country and the NHS increased its efforts to cope with large numbers of testing required in its hospitals. As far as community testing was concerned, it was said that about 2,000 tests a day could be carried out by local public-health organisations to be processed in PHE's Colindale laboratory, with results promised in 24 hours. 10,000 a day would need to be carried out soon. These were moderately high numbers and testing protocols restricted which symptoms permitted a patient to be tested. Bahrain with only 1.5 million inhabitants was to test 900,000 people, or an average of 6,000 a day every date for five months.

Whitehall's messaging was meanwhile becoming chaotic and deadly. On the backfoot after Johnson pumping hands, the government geared up to tell people how to 'social distance' to fight spread of the disease. Belatedly alternatives to shaking hands and advice on standing further apart were reported to be being tested.

108

Dr Jenny Harries, one of England's Deputy Chief Medical Officers, who would soon become a regular media fixture, and a controversial figure, went on the record as saying that the peak of the British outbreak was expected to start within the next fortnight, 'when we will be likely to advise people with symptoms to self-isolate and we expect the start of the peak to come within that period'. Dr Harries' statements were presumably informed by one or other of the competing sets of epidemiological modellers at Imperial College, The London School of Hygiene and Tropical Medicine, and Oxford University. Pushing back against Harries, public-health Professor Paul Hunter suggested that hundreds of cases were already undiagnosed, that 'if it is spreading in the community, it will spread. The only uncertainty is how quickly it takes off and when the peak is'. Given what became known later about the holes in the government testing protocols, Professor Hunter seemed a lot closer to the mark.

At this point SAGE, the Scientific Advisory Group on Emergencies, the COBR for scientists, which provided advice to government and would become a major focus of criticism, made a prominent appearance. It intervened on behalf of the government on the hot topics of cancelling mass gatherings and self-isolation of those with 'flu-like symptoms. SAGE confidently claimed that 'plans by other countries to ban mass gatherings were counter-productive'.

How SAGE might have come to this conclusion was difficult to fathom. Not for nothing have many of the worse infectious disease threats been known as crowd diseases. During the 1849 cholera epidemic in Liverpool, Medical Officer of Health William Duncan argued that what killed over 5,000 people that summer was being spread as people lived crammed together, cheek by jowl, in the city's slums. Overcrowding in the American military cantonments in 1919 seems to have created the ideal conditions for Influenza to incubate and thrive. Following the enormous street festival in Philadelphia that September, with the 'flu virus circulating freely, people began to die in their hundreds within days.

SAGE appeared to have been advised by David Halpern, head of the government Behavioural Insights Team or 'nudge unit'. His main concern was absenteeism from work. He worried that advice to people to stay at home if they had 'flu-like symptoms might be used as an excuse to avoid work. Halpern was reported as arguing against early intervention on the grounds of not 'crying wolf'. In particular, he said, 'if you go too early and tell people to take a week off work when they have coronavirus, and then a couple of weeks later they have another cough, it's likely they'll say "come on already" [if told to stay home again].'

Professor Neil Ferguson, leader of the Imperial College team of modellers advising the government, was later to comment, 'the issue is that people spend a very small amount of time during the week at a mass gathering. It is not that mass gatherings don't contribute at all [to the spread of a virus] but at a population level, stopping them has a marginal impact'. He added that some people will get infected but that stopping sporting events 'would not have had a major impact on the spread of the epidemic'.

To many race-goers and football supporters, familiar with the cultures of their favourite sports and the extensive socialisation involved, this would seem doubtful. Ferguson's peers were even more bemused. 'Even the use of the toilets at a mass event should be seen as a fantastic opportunity' for an unknown virus to spread, observed one NHS statistician.

David Nunan and John Brassey of the Nuffield Centre for Evidence-Based Medicine, Oxford University, did a review of the scholarly studies on the subject. They concluded, 'The effect of restricting and cancelling mass gatherings and sporting events on infectious diseases is poorly established and requires further assessment. The best-available evidence suggests multiple-day events with crowded communal accommodations are most associated with increased risk.' The two scholars published their conclusions on 20 March, but presumably Professor Ferguson and others at SAGE had gone through the same literature. So how did they reach the conclusion on which they based their advice to the government and dismissed the impact of mass gatherings as 'marginal'?

Experts in other countries weren't second guessing COVID. They had already intervened to stop sporting events, including Italy where football matches were being played behind closed doors, Bahrain had cancelled the Formula 1 races, and the July Tokyo Olympics were in doubt. In California, the famous Coachella arts and music festival was postponed.

The tally of avoidable deaths was taking off. Boris Johnson's cabinet was putting people in Britain in harm's way and some of those were going to die.

11

Left to Die, 'Herd Immunity'

'Fantastic afternoon at Twickenham', Boris Johnson gushed on his Facebook page on 7 March, with a picture of the massive crowd at the Rugby and a cheek-by-jowl group photo of him in the middle of the attractive Red Roses women's team. Public-health estimates were that being within two metres of a carrier was a risk. Nonetheless, the advice to the government was, apparently from the Chief Scientific Adviser Sir Patrick Vallance, that attendance at events such as Johnson's and the four-day race meeting at Cheltenham, two concerts in Bristol by the Stereophonics and the European Championship semi-final football match at Anfield between Liverpool and Atletico Madrid should go ahead.

Fans needed no encouragement. Hundreds of thousands of race goers from around the country and beyond attended the four day meeting in Cheltenham beginning on Tuesday 10 March. Furthermore, 3,000 Atletico supporters made the journey from Madrid, a city under COVID siege, to spend 24 hours on Merseyside on March 11.

During a fireside chat that was broadcast on Johnson's Facebook page, released on the same day, Deputy Chief Medical Officer Dr Harries, explained why Britain was so different.

'In this country', Dr Harries said, 'we have expert modellers looking at what we think will happen with the virus, big gatherings are not seen to be something which is going to have a big effect.'

What defines 'a big effect'? From Monday's rugby match to Tuesday's fireside chat, the number of known cases had quintupled. Three weeks later distinctive spikes of deaths appeared in the hospitals around Cheltenham and on Merseyside. A physician in Ireland was to comment that half of his first batch of Corona patients in intensive care had travelled to Cheltenham's to attend the races. But by then a panicked Johnson cabinet had locked down the country *en masse* and revised its point of view— it now even considered 1-1 contacts in shops, restaurants and offices as having an effect big enough to require its intervention, never mind big gatherings.

There was news that the local Cheltenham MP Alex Chalk had received substantial horse-racing hospitality and that health secretary Matt Hancock, MP for Newmarket, had received substantial political donations from the horse racing industry. Amid allegations that betting-industry money had played a part in enabling the races to go ahead, the recriminations began.

Arriving back home on 11 March and digesting the news, I made the difficult decision not to go to the match at Anfield that evening. With the Johnson cabinet at odds with most governments around the world, except Donald Trump, the media was again casting around to speak to public-health experts who weren't muzzled by political advisors or ministers and could cast light on the confusing mixed messages from Whitehall.

Speaking later to the *Daily Telegraph*, I explained my position that 'bringing 3,000 supporters from a very-high incidence area was basically just wrong, and the view that open-air events don't pose a threat is really simplistic. I hope I'm wrong but I believe that people were put in harm's way that night'.

That evening, I received a call from the BBC in Manchester to be on Newsnight later on in the evening. My comments bear inclusion here:

We've got a complacent attitude… we've wasted a month when we should have been engaging with the public… if this now spreads the way it looks as though it's going to spread, there will not be enough hospital beds and people will have to be nursed at home… we should have got a grip on this a month ago…. I want to know why we are not testing, why we haven't tested those people coming back from Italy and are now amongst us? We've got a recipe for community-spread here.

The following day, March 12, with the numbers of infected people rising inexorably, the government issued its bombshell announcement that it was stopping community testing for COVID-19 and was instead concentrating on testing those in hospitals. The government dropped the 'contain' phase and moved to the 'delay' phase of the Johnson-Whitty plan. Defending the decision, Deputy Chief Medical Officer Dr Jennie Harries explained that at that stage community testing was 'not an appropriate intervention'.

If this had been an enemy attack instead of an attack by a virus, the equivalent announcement would have been that troops would hereafter withdraw from the streets of Stalingrad and that the fight would be limited to the hospitals where victims were being brought in. There would be no scouting the slightest enemy movements. There would be no door-to-door battle to rout the enemy. No one would try to capture the enemy to stop clusters of death forming. How that was 'appropriate' as a matter of public health was not easy to understand.

Later, at a hearing of the Health Select Committee on 5 May, Harries was to change this brazen government statement and finally admitted that the problem with testing came down to the question 'what capacity do we have'. Dr Harries also conceded that there was a follow-up bottle neck with 'the ongoing support beyond that'. After centrally hogging decisions for a month and a half, Johnson's cabinet had managed to gouge out Britain's eyes as to where COVID was striking until its worst-affected patients finally admitted themselves to a nearby hospital. Whereas health officers were able to intercept the virus locally in Bahrain's four municipalities, their equivalents in Britain's regions and areas were now fully blinded, as was Whitehall.

From that day, there was not much left that stood in the way of COVID's potential for infecting new carriers. Sight of the virus would not be recovered for the duration of the lockdown with an attendant rise in avoidable casualties as a result of the decisions made by Johnson's cabinet. It is hard to exaggerate the importance of what had befallen—for want of a better word—Britain. Bahrain would not have been able to achieve its WHO world rank without tracing and testing, the spinal column of public health.

Dr Harries was merely another British scientists who put their professional reputation close to the firing line with words such as the one above. Given the gravity of the situation, it begged the question why government experts were behaving like this?

A likely seed for this unusual situation was sown on 2 January by Dominic Cummings. In a bookend to Johnson's war on the BBC, he declared war on civil-service mandarins on his blog. He wanted 'super-talented weirdos' who brought 'genuine cognitive diversity'. The message, amplified as the months went on, was received loud and clear in Whitehall. Stick your head above the parapet and the two leading men in No 10 would chop it off. Indeed this was to happen with the rare civil servant who dared to offered mild 'cognitively-diverse' push-back to No 10's opinions. As the 2013 PHE reforms had muzzled the local Public Health Directors, Cummings's 2020 Whitehall reform-threat was gagging the top of the civil service—even before they spoke. 'As you wish, Sir', was what the Johnson-Cummings tandem wanted. Anything less would unleash media leaks that killed by a thousand rumours, as reportedly claimed by top civil servants.

Having Johnson's ear, Cummings succeeded in surrounding No 10 with a donut of top-civil servants and experts terrified to contradict them. Unless they happened to be 'misfits with odd skills', of course—another desirable qualification cited by Cummings in January, though admittedly one unlikely to land you a top civil-service job which required more ordinary skills. Like all Catch-22s, it had been an authoritarian move. Cummings's weirdoes weren't there to question what the two ancient-history Oxford graduates had already decided for themselves. It was merely about bits left blank on their road map for five years of unchallenged government, the blue sky they hadn't looked at yet.

Even the warning shot in late January by Johnson and Cummings's own social-media-guru Craig Dillon, clearly a capable expert on what mattered to the British population, fell well outside No 10's brand new tent. He wasn't even an Oxbridge English graduate who chats 'about Lacan at dinner parties', another type loathed by Cummings, as vented on 2 January. On the one hand, the French psychoanalyst Lacan was a foreigner popular in British academia for a brand of feminism and lefty sexual-identity thinking, and on the other Michael Gove and Johnson's special political adviser Munira Mirza were both Oxford English-graduates, with Gove quoting tropes by Italian Marxist Antonio Gramsci.

None of this cultural hinterland wove through Dillon though. He was a journalism graduate from the University of Westminster, an institution that had started life as a polytechnic. On 2 January, Cummings had also detailed that he was looking for communications experts who didn't do 'talking to the lobby'. But the net result was still that you might as well talk to the hand. Cummings's ideas weren't so much open for discussion as closed like a narrow one-way street with a tight seal at its entrance. All cars were red—unless Cummings happened to be looking for another colour.

Boris Johnson's tone changed dramatically from its previous bouncy abandon. Speaking after a meeting of COBR, he dropped the florid language and starkly warned that 'many more people will lose loved ones to coronavirus'. Gone was the chirpy 50's public announcement-style suggestion that everything was all right and that Britain should sing 'Happy Birthday' twice to save itself from the virus while washing hands. For the public it was another sudden change to interpret, but at least the prime minister was starting to show an understanding of the crisis that was looming.

That evening of Tuesday March 12, I found myself on the BBC Question Time panel from West Bromwich in the Midlands, facing government treasury spokesman, Steve Barclay. Fresh back from Bahrain, where I had witnessed first-hand, first-class proactive leadership and a systematic public-health approach that was already demonstrating its effectiveness, my sense of frustration at a government unwilling to offer leadership and a public-health system in chaos was only too apparent. The chair of the programme, Fiona Bruce, was not best pleased. She summarised, 'John, you are a reasonably lone voice on the panel, I'm not passing judgement'. Arguably that was the sort of thing Cummings was looking for—I attended Newcastle University Medical School and the University of London's School of Hygiene and Tropical Medicine—but I doubt that he paid any attention.

Confused by the COVID world news and the vacillating government statements that weren't adding up, panic was spreading around Britain. By the end of the day mortgage companies had announced payment holidays, amid reports of panic buying in the shops, not least for lavatory rolls, as if people were expecting a siege. It also transpired that the NHS 111 online service had been giving out wrong advice to visitors returning from Italy, namely that they had no need to self-isolate in contradiction to PHE advice that they should stay at home for 14 days, regardless of whether they felt unwell. Meanwhile the Queen had

117

begun to make a point of not shaking hands in audiences at Buckingham Palace.

On Friday 13 March the UK woke to find itself in a new and confusing situation. Overnight the Chief Medical Officer's original 4-point plan seemed to have flipped into a one-point plan, 'Herd Immunity'. Out of the blue, the Chief Scientific Adviser appeared to float the idea of letting the virus run its course, with the aim of achieving herd immunity rather than containing the epidemic.

The usual meaning of the term herd immunity, as used by public-health practitioners, is the attainment of a sufficient level of population immunity as to confer a collective 'herd' level of protection, such that an infectious agent cannot find enough people or animals who are susceptible to infection to propagate itself. This prevents virus-spread from taking off exponentially even if the infectious agent is around in the environment. It is the point of vaccinating young children against the historically serious viral illnesses of measles, mumps and rubella (German measles) with MMR.

An instant controversy erupted when the Chief Scientific Adviser, Sir Patrick Vallance, seemed to advocate that about 60%, or 40 million people, would need to catch the coronavirus to build up 'herd immunity'. In the case of MMR the aim is to achieve 95% of each cohort of children being vaccinated to create herd immunity for the population. On the face of it, the 60% seemed very low indeed. In addition, Sir Patrick advanced this figure about a new virus whose behaviour was still pretty much unknown after western scientists first set eyes on it a few months earlier.

Where did all this knowledge come from? Sir Patrick offered no detailed explanation. He said on Sky News, 'Well, we've got a panel of very experienced scientists'.

His was not the first sign that No 10, seemed to think herd immunity was the new plan. Two days before her fireside chat with Johnson, Dr Harries had on Monday March 9 defended that schools stayed open (only for them to be closed 'indefinitely' over a week later in dramatic fashion). Dr Harries argued on the Today Programme, 'If you have a new disease, the normal thing is, it will take off gradually. It will rise very rapidly at one point and come back down again when it effectively runs out of people in the population to infect.' If that statement were applied to HIV, the world would still be waiting for the virus to run out of people to infect. In the case of the seasonal 'flu, it was also an outlier statement that strained at the seams.

Presumably, the 'experienced scientists' Sir Patrick referred to were statisticians, or in Dr Harries's words at her fireside chat, 'expert modellers'. Any statistical analysis is only as good as the raw data inputted or else it is a case of GIGO, or 'Garbage In Garbage Out'. Dr Harries made a point of distinguishing 'our' team from those across our borders.

So in what shape was Britain's raw data? At this stage, the only hard UK facts available to scientists were the virus tests that had been carried out in the UK. At the first sighting of herd immunity on Monday's Today Programme, there were 374 confirmed COVID cases in the UK. But, No 10 knew this was really the tip of an iceberg of infections. Three days later Dr Harries would announce the shut-down Whitehall's community testing and track-tracing programme for capacity reasons.

The absence of reliable raw data was an ancillary cost of Britain's reluctant testing and tracing of carriers in January, February and March when numbers were low. Unlike Bahrain and other countries that had made the organisation of maximum testing capacity from the start a top priority to locate at an early stage all infections on the map, the UK had none of this. By Friday March 13 there was a low number of virus tests that made up the raw data for government epidemiologists. In addition, there was no reliable data on regional and local variation, nor the ability to drill down to neighbourhood and postcode levels. If Vallance's

60% herd immunity for the new disease was based on this data set, it wasn't exactly a reliable figure to pin your hopes on, let alone the health of the population in England and Wales.

In an interview with the BBC, Sir Patrick had added 'our aim is to try to reduce the peak (of the epidemic curve), not suppress it completely; also, because the vast majority of people get a mild illness, to build up some kind of herd immunity so more people are immune to this disease and we reduce the transmission, at the same time we protect those who are most vulnerable to it'. Dr Harries, in her fireside chat with Johnson on the Wednesday had also called it 'push the peak of the epidemic forward'.

But with what exactly?

After admitting defeat on community testing and contact-tracing of those connected to a death or infection, all that the government was left with was giving the population advice to self-isolate, to wash your hands frequently and shop for the elderly. How did that add up to Johnson's aim that his government 'suppress' and 'push the peak forward' in the words of the Chief Scientific Adviser but also the Deputy Medical Officer in her fireside chat with the prime minister. In practise, it seemed clear that the cabinet's view was that, as far as they were concerned, nothing would be placed in between the population and COVID.

The row built over the weekend as the ethical implications became clear of allowing the virus to run its course rather than trying to eliminate it. Johnson spoke of 'taking it on the chin' (he himself would come perilously close to paying the price for the nationwide policy chopped and changed for others).

Dizzy from government officials' pirouettes, the population's panic grew. By now it had become clear that the gradient of the UK epidemic curve, far from being gentler than the terrifying graphs from Italy where deaths had risen to 1,016 in the previous day, an increase of 50% in 24 hours, was actually similar. If anything, it was steeper. Britain's reported death toll had doubled in two days and was already on a trajectory to continue at the same pace.

What the Chief Scientific Adviser's discussion of herd immunity certainly did was offer a distraction. Coming the day after the collapse of the Johnson-Whitty 'contain, delay, research and mitigate' strategy, it created a lot of heated debate about morality that absorbed the media's attention. Instead of calling Johnson on his government's catastrophic failure to deliver, the newspapers and broadcasters sank their teeth into this novel bone of contention.

At the same time, by mooting replacement with an early nineteenth-century style *laissez-faire* strategy, Johnson created the rhetorical illusion that his cabinet had so far done more than what needed to be done. The end of community testing wasn't a major public-health failure so much as a liberal government saying goodbye to an excess piece of luggage. It was also a campaign of subtle self-congratulation for having tried at least.

Unless of course, you were aware of 175 years of public-health history. In that case you understood Whitehall to be informing Britain that the Johnson government was going to leave people to die except if they were to reach an NHS hospital in time. On what we knew so far about the virus, by that time it would be too late for most victims from the clinical evidence that had been flooding in from hospitals in Britain and elsewhere. The people were as much patients as test cases how best to fight the novel disease that was attacking their bodies. Waiting for 'herd immunity' was nigh the equivalent of the social killing of those most susceptible to the virus in Britain: the aged and those weakened by chronic ailments, as well as a minority of others of all age groups, including the young, who drew the short straw for as yet unknown reasons.

The following weekend Tim Shipman in the *Sunday Times* would report that Michael Gove said that he had come to the view that 'we need to run it hot'. 'Hot' being the deaths of some of the people who helped pay for his ministerial post, car and chauffeur in the fair expectation that the government would govern. Even if one thought such ethics were for snowflakes, was this letting the chips-fall-where-they-may strategy acceptable from a cabinet that had clamoured to be 'very well prepared'? Had that meant no more than that it was well-prepared to sit on its hands?

It was more likely an opportunistic media strategy designed to cover up Johnson's failure to engage so far. Similar media pyrotechnics would be deployed for the duration of the lockdown and after, only to be overtaken by the facts. By August, Britain would have the highest number of COVID deaths per million people in the entire world as a result of Johnson's handling of the pandemic. Only Belgium had a higher figure—a result, Belgium said, because it included in its figures deaths in care homes where staff had a mere suspicion that they were COVID-related whereas other countries merely tallied proven COVID deaths.

The media smelled a rat behind the flip-flopping cabinet, despite the Chief Scientific Adviser's words after Dr Harries's bombshell. It kept looking for alternative authorities to make sense of what was really happening.

As an English expert advising Bahrain, I was in demand as such an alternative authority. Where the British government was forever shape-shifting, the island country was showing COVID result after result, soberly and without jokes, providing facts rather than bloated intentions.

The following evening, I was invited on Channel 4 News with Matt Frei where I again criticised the government response, saying that we were in a grave situation, only a couple of weeks behind Italy, that we had failed to test systematically, to engage with the public and to mobilise the community. In response, Dr Clare Gerada, formerly Chair of the Royal College of General Practitioners, said that she was glad that I was not leading COBR instead of Johnson. According to Dr Gerada, I was ill-informed.

On Friday 13 March, Sir Patrick also told Sky News, 'If you completely locked down absolutely everything, probably for a period of four months or more, then you would suppress this virus.'

A lockdown wasn't, however, what the government wanted, said Sir Patrick. He explained the reasoning behind not shutting the borders like Italy had done on 9 March. 'It is the case of course that all of the evidence from previous epidemics suggests that when you do that... you get the second peak'. What, Sir Patrick reaffirmed on Sky, the Johnson cabinet wanted was to 'allow enough of us who are going to get mild illness to become immune to this to help with the sort of whole population response which would protect everybody'.

Just to make it clear to experts and the public alike, Sir Patrick nailed his colours to the mast with regards to what he said about COVID, herd immunity, and lockdown. He stated unequivocally, 'My job as Chief Scientific Adviser is to speak scientific truth to power and that's exactly what I will do.'

Finally chairing the COBR meetings on COVID, Johnson was to make yet another flipflop in a matter of days.

12

Chickens Coming Home to Roost

For the want of a nail, the shoe was lost;
For the want of the shoe, the horse was lost;
For the want of the horse, the rider was lost;
For the want of the rider, the battle was lost;
For the want of the battle, the kingdom was lost;
And all from the want of a horseshoe nail.

On the same day Britain's Chief Scientific Adviser mooted herd immunity from nowhere, the WHO issued its guidance through Dr Tedros: 'You must take a comprehensive approach.' 'Not Testing Alone.' 'Not Contact Tracing Alone.' 'Not Quarantine Alone.' 'Not Social Distancing Alone.' 'Do It All!' The WHO had been very clear from early on in the pandemic that according to the consensus opinion of its experts the key to COVID containment was testing, contact tracing, and isolating those affected.

Dr Tedros's guidance wasn't going to cost him his WHO job. His adamant (and often repeated) advice was the opposite of controversial. WHO's approach to containing outbreaks and epidemics had been fundamental to the effective practice of public-health for centuries, the identification, isolation and quarantining of cases predating the ability to test for causal agents. What would, however, have cost him his job was if he advocated a return to the nineteenth century and advised global governments to wait for herd immunity to establish itself and allow the new virus to strike its victims wherever and whenever.

The proof of the pudding is in the eating. One of the characteristics of most countries that dealt successfully with COVID-19 is that they acted promptly, vigorously, and effectively by identifying and isolating new cases of infection. This included China, after the initial epidemic, Hong Kong, South Korea, Taiwan, New Zealand and Australia, Germany, Denmark, Finland, Norway and Cuba. Their core technique was little different from the one that Liverpool's Dr William Duncan and London's Dr John Snow used almost two centuries ago.

But you didn't even have to go that far abroad, or back in history, for success. In Wales Ceredigion County Council, which covers the University of Aberystwyth, ordered its own low-cost community tracing. It was a remarkable repeat from the time Liverpool Town Council funded Dr Duncan's post as the world's first Medical Officer of Health in 1847. When the council's Chief Executive Eifion Evans said at a Gold Command meeting about COVID, the council's equivalent of COBR, 'are we missing a trick?', his deputy Barry Rees, a former biology teacher of 16 years, pointed out that contract-tracing is standard in case of outbreaks of *legionnaires* disease and in South East Asian countries that had borne the brunt of previous coronavirus attacks.

At this meeting, Rees suggested to his executive director and to Plaid Cymru Leader of the Council Ellen ap Gwynn that Ceredigion should be 'pursuing the disease rather than following it'. With their assent he project-managed a team pulled together from relevant departments. Further to Rees's research on google to see what other countries were doing, he set up their feet-on-the-ground contact-tracing team with Ceredigion's manager for public protection. One of the county council's partnerships included a Public Health Director who was the point of contact for notifiable outbreaks. She reported with one other manager to the executive social-care director in a team funded by Public Health Wales, the Welsh equivalent of Public Health England.

The case of Ceredigion, population 75,000, spoke for itself. Using the council's in-house expertise Rees set up a budget-neutral paperless tracking system that conformed to the rules on data protection and good governance. The county was not only well-ahead of Whitehall's roll out of a national test, track and trace-system, but also of its first case of COVID. In a carbon copy of Bahrain, in fact, Rees's team was up and running to contact-trace every single confirmed case from the start. Anyone contacted was given very detailed instructions on what they must do to keep others safe from virus spread. Rees also instructed his team to check up on a council staff reporting sick to avoid institutional spread.

Even at this micro level, and incredibly early on, Rees ran into the same problems that caused the Whitehall PHE/PHW community-tracing system to self-immolate on 12 March. The failure was to blind the whole of Britain to the virus's points of attack around the country, except in Ceredigion County. As it had its own low-cost programme, it carried on contact-tracing as before whenever there was a suspected case in the county.

Very early on Rees had dropped reliance on positive testing results because the minimum of 48 hours to get test results back could mean that the virus had bolted well before a case was confirmed. Instead he relied on the presumption of COVID in case of symptoms, reckoning that early prevention was more effective than a bull's eye that was too late. 'The system could fail because of the numbers involved', Rees said. Test results were part of the programme's feedback loop and were fed into a detailed data chart of the enemy virus's hide-outs in Rees's territory.

Ceredigion didn't just have its own community tracking system. The political leadership of the county and its civil service top were on COVID tenterhooks well-before Boris Johnson was. They knew that at Easter the county's caravan sites and second-homes and hotels would fill up and its population balloon. While the national government ignored these holiday migrations—not 'a big effect' according to Dr Harries, Deputy Chief Medical Officer, on 11 March—Ceredigion's leaders did not agree. The county council also liaised with Aberystwyth University, one of the first universities to close in the country.

The results for Ceredigion are almost hard to believe and are among the very lowest in the UK. Only the Isles of Scilly, with a population of 2153 in the middle of the Celtic Sea recorded fewer COVID deaths. Ceredigion's outcomes were even more impressive when compared to the neighbouring county of Powys with its lower density and smaller towns, compared with Ceredigion's university town of Aberystwyth. As of June 24th the mortality rate from COVID-19 in Ceredigion was 9.6 per 100,000 whereas that for Powys was 68.7.

Public Health Wales held back a per-county breakdown of Wales's officially-reported COVID deaths. But when ONS calculated excess deaths by county Powys County Council published them on its website as a public record for its population. On the difference between the two counties, Dr Giri Shankar of PHW observed that in Wales, 'The pandemic progressed predominantly East to West'. But Aberystwyth is reached by the A44, the major road that bisects both Ceredigion and Powys from East to West and it is not easy to see how the virus's East-West vector was a major reason in Ceredigion's impressive results. Did those who were infected make U-turns upon reaching the Ceredigion border?

On 7 May, the Johnson cabinet would announce a new venture: the £10 billion 'cross-government' Test & Trace organisation headed by former TalkTalk CEO and amateur jockey Baroness Dido Harding. Community testing 2.0, the London-led programme was to deploy the army, Amazon, and a cascade of commercial subcontractors who were to guarantee up to 25,000 employees. Test & Trace was to shrivel to 12,000 employees a few months later, subject to service contracts that had been signed by the government. On 12 August, Leicester and Luton local councils, using council tax bills, welfare support bills and shoe-leather while knocking on doors, would report a success rate of 80% in tracking contacts of a local COVID flare-up within 48 hours, the minimum required to be effective according to SAGE, as reported in *The Times*. Test & Trace systems did not record or provide information conforming to SAGE's advice the paper observed. Local authorities were denied additional money by the cabinet and instead it appointed Baroness Harding on 18 August as head of the National Institute for Health Protection, the name that replaced PHE and Test & Trace.

What could you achieve if you were to combine Ceredigion's low-cost hands-on nineteenth-century-style, almost paperclip and rubber-band (Rees had put together a database) local community contact-tracing with state-of-the-art testing capabilities while scaling up the population by a factor ten?

Enter Alex Friedrich, head of infection control in Groningen county in the North Netherlands an area 50% larger than Ceredigion with a total population of 600,000 and a university town like Aberystwyth, but with a much larger population of 200,000.

Friedrich, decided to follow the WHO's instruction to test not only severe and priority cases, but everyone in order to contain the disease. In fact, his was, in theory, Britain's approach as well, until Dr Harries announced that Britain threw in the towel on 12 March. Friedrich told journalist Naomi O'Leary, 'You save lives by doing diagnostics. Proper diagnostics, case tracing, information, is one of the strongest weapons we have to fight the virus.'

Like Rees in Ceredigion, Friedrich had the authority to project-manage his own public-health efforts. Instead of a biology teacher, he had the advantage of being professor of virology at Groningen University. There was no reliable literature on COVID-19 since its first appearance in January. He knew however that coronaviruses regularly affected livestock and called vets in the area to create a model. He also picked up the phone to call colleagues in Rome where the first European cases had been. 'We can't accept that people will all get infected... It's just the consequences of our insufficient action to protect people', he told O'Leary.

He struck further unpublished epidemiological gold with the Italians. 'The Italians were the best in publishing on a database all the data on a very regional and provincial level. They gave to us how many healthcare workers were infected, how many people were infected. That's impressive how Italians did this, we really learned from them. I was able to compare it and say oh my god, that's a very different infection from other infections. We really owe a lot to them.'

Like Rees he didn't get any extra budget. But Friedrich's 600 plus colleagues of his university's antibiotic-resistance network agreed to help him out. Friedrich also knew that testing was a game-changer. 'Ten years ago we did not have such rapid diagnostic tools, you might have had a diagnosis in ten days or five, now within a few hours you have a result. This is so strong.'

He organised a make-shift laboratory tent on the university campus where he could do his own immediate testing within a protected environment for those doing the testing. The only real logistical bottle neck he had were the swabs, where would he get supplies from and who would take them—which is where his students came in. They were sitting at home doing nothing and gladly agreed to help out to learn something.

As of August 5, Groningen's public-health department (GGD) reported 17 deaths as a result of Corona. A remarkable result achieved with very little except a determination of local health officers and volunteers to protect their population. Neither

Ceredigion nor Groningen had the budget to put together a state-of-the-art War Room with live feeds and a foreign public-health consultant as Bahrain had. Their governments hadn't authorised central support and the additional budget to do so that the King of Bahrain had granted. But Rees's and Friedrich's results held up well.

In the British Isles, incidentally, there was a local government that, like the Bahrain government, had the independent means to invest in the protection of its population. On the Isle of Mann the local government initially sent specimens for testing to the UK. But it abandoned this when it noticed, like Barry Rees in Ceredigion, that it all took too long and was inadequate. Not having to answer to Whitehall, the island bought a second-hand PCR machine of their own and conducted extensive test analysis at their own laboratories in the hospital in Douglas. After this change, the numbers of new infections declined sharply and deaths flatlined with a total of 24 in a population of 85,000 by the summer. Given the false start, it compared well to the 8 deaths in Ceredigion (as of June) with roughly the same size population.

Liverpool City Region, with a population as great as Bahrain's, recorded more than 1500 deaths according to the *Liverpool Echo* of 17 June. Bahrain, with no general lockdown, tallied 130 deaths by July, while in Liverpool public-health officials had to wait for and follow instructions from London on what to do and not to do in their area.

Unlike Barry Rees, Professor Friedrich and Crown Prince Salman, from January, Whitehall's central instruction to its public-health employees around Britain's localities was marked by tentativeness and procrastination while the cabinet remained in limbo. Whether it was testing, tracing and isolating, home working, school and university closures, suspension of mass gatherings and flights, the usual line to take seemed to be, 'we may have to think about that, it wouldn't work here, or it will make matters worse'.

Dominic Cummings' call for civil-service outsiders included 'great project managers'. But would he have been interested to hear what Barry Rees, Alex Friedrich, Prince Salman, or the Isle of Man government had to say about how to project manage routing the virus with minimal damaging to the local economy?

Cummings was right about one thing. Whitehall was the old buffer in a London club, hogging decisions and information while doing nothing of substance. But Cummings and Johnson were cut from the same London cloth. Unlike Rees, Friedrich and Prince Salman, Cummings clearly had no interest in taking inventory of what expertise he already had among the 423,050 government employees Johnson commanded in March 2020. The three were capable professionals passionate about doing their job well. Barry Rees, like Wiltshire Public Health Director Daszkiewicz did not seek the limelight. Like Cummings he called himself an 'ideas man' when interviewed, but in a self-denigrating way in his one interview in the Welsh media. He stressed the invaluable help of his colleagues who rose to the occasion. He did not think the grass was greener elsewhere. He understood what resources he had and made use of them—unlike No 10.

Johnson's acquiescence to the end of community testing in Britain on 12 March and to the sole concentration of whatever testing capacity there was on confirming the diagnosis of hospital cases of the virus would have far-reaching consequences. For the sake of those who lost relatives, their health, or would lose their livelihoods after the end of Rishi Sunak's lockdown furlough scheme in October, it was worth taking stock of where the UK found itself after Dr Harries set off the government's bombshell on 12 March.

There was no longer a chance, for example, to intercept 'super-spreaders', the phenomenon that every so often a single infected person will set off a tsunami of infections around them. It also meant that frontline clinical staff as well as a wide range of essential workers, including bus and taxi drivers, together with public facing shop workers and operatives in risky trades such as slaughterhouses and meat processing plants went unprotected; and it meant that those to be found in 'Petri-dish' settings like the Princess Diamond, including workers and the resident population in care homes and prisons, remained unprotected and in harm's way.

Falling back on NHS hospitals had its own price. The top political priority of avoiding the embarrassment of hospitals being unable to cope with the numbers of cases coming through the doors, led to the discharge of thousands of untested frail and elderly patients into care homes that were without tests or Personal Protective Equipment (PPE) and ill-prepared for what they faced. Given the limitations of the testing protocols mandated by London, patients with COVID but without the required symptoms would have been among them. The result was the ignition of a parallel epidemic to that in the community and in the hospitals which would eventually be responsible for thousands of avoidable premature deaths from COVID-19.

One of the few successful central measures taken by the government was to move thousands of homeless rough sleepers off the streets and into hotels for the duration, with apparently significant benefits to their mental and physical health. Other marginal groups such as sex-workers, however, were simply ignored.

Inexplicably, given the results *vis-a-vis* rough-sleepers, this billeting approach was not rolled out further to key segments of the population who were both pivotal to social care and could, because of their job, inadvertently become super spreaders. Billeting NHS and care-home staff in hotels, boarding houses, student accommodation would have created a quarantine ring around vulnerable older people or those with pre-existing conditions with regular testing of those billeted, protecting both them and those in their care. None of this happened. Why?

Testing

What were the issues behind the lack of testing capacity that the government admitted to? The UK was not the only country facing capacity issues as the epidemic struck. PCR (Polymerase Chain Reaction) test machines were essential, together with the swabs to take samples from the nose and throat, together with the reagents and enzymes to amplify segments of RNA (Ribonucleic acid) for analysis to positively identify the virus. The main manufacturers of PCR machines were in Germany, Switzerland and the US and the need to increase the numbers of these machines, together with a shortage of reagents, enzymes and swabs was what lay behind the embarrassing situation that the UK found itself in.

This was coupled with the progressive reduction of laboratory facilities that was a part of a ten year long process driven by an ideology of economies of scale, outsourcing and centralising into London and the South-East. The regionally based Public Health Service that had been folded into the Health Protection Agency in 2003 had been followed by a withering away of local laboratory capacity, something that had been consolidated initially with the abolition of the Regional Health Authorities who had reported directly to the Chief Medical Officer rather than to a separate body in Whitehall.

By 2020 the first port of call by Public Health England was confined to the laboratories at Colindale in North London. As did Barry Rees, PHE must have known that Colindale's testing capacity was going to be swamped in a matter of time. The failure of PHE to mobilise the remaining NHS capacity from around the country, as well as the extensive capacity to be found in university laboratories, until late in the day remained a mystery, particularly given the mouthing of Johnson and his ministers that they were 'well-prepared'.

The explanation given for shortages of reagents was that this was not a UK strength, despite having a vibrant pharmaceutical manufacturing sector. But, in view of Professor Friedrich's tent laboratory, it didn't require a lot of strength just the art of persuasion in seeking cooperation to address an emergency. What the cabinet may have meant to say is that, unlike local organisations, it didn't have a clue where excess capacity was up and down the country, and nor did it have the social network to arrange for it to be activated, let alone did it have the manpower to project-manage such a task centrally and in a very short time frame from London.

Comparisons with Germany, whose federal structure had enabled it to maintain a resilient regional network of collaborating laboratories highlighted the disastrous effects of the incessant drive to centralisation in the UK. Although the German local public-health system had also suffered from a lack of attention before the pandemic, a concerted drive to build local capacity for the leg work of testing and tracing had saved the day. This had enabled Germany to reach daily levels of testing that the UK could only fantasise about. The distressing position the UK found itself in was exacerbated by the refusal to participate in EU wide procurement of hard and software as well as PPE in the early days of February, a manifestation of the politics of Brexit.

Unlike Professor Friedrich, Whitehall was uninterested to 'call a friend' and to adopt practices from elsewhere. It seemed as if only researchers who spoke and wrote English and worked in Britain were worth taking into account when assessing COVID. When it came to a light-footed response to novel challenges, the 'not invented here' issue was a familiar one to those working in the public services and in public health. Painstaking networking, coalition building and persuasive advocacy was essential if innovation and diffusion of best practice was to be achieved. This kind of *modus operandi* is bread and butter to local authorities and their partner agencies from small authorities such as Ceredigion to the largest in the country. It is, however, alien to the tribal warfare between departments in Whitehall where mandarins keep a beady eye on the slices of budget that might be raided by one of their colleagues in order to feather their portfolios of responsibilities.

In recent decades the popular-free market belief that these goals were more attainable through market mechanisms had grown across the political spectrum. Future historians might well reflect also on the well-rehearsed personality characteristics of Boris Johnson, whose combination of laziness and unwillingness to accept responsibility for decisions in his personal and professional life, together with a belief in the free market offering solutions to social questions, was well chronicled.

Johnson's cabinet pretended on Friday 13 March that it was going to rely on herd immunity, but in reality it knew it had lost the first battle with the virus. There was still time however. What was obvious was that Whitehall's organisation was designed to act adequately in the case of a terrorist accident, such as the Skripal attack in Salisbury or *legionnaires* disease, but that it was incapable of dealing with a stealth attack such as a pandemic. However, at this crucial moment Johnson remained distracted. Dominic Cummings, for his part, was busy subjugating Whitehall's civil-service top and ministers' special political advisers to his rule while repressing any sign of dissension. And so the hot potato went round and round, as no one fancied being the bearer of bad news to the two men. It was ironic no one dared to be Cassandra in the presence of the two self-congratulatory ancient-history graduates.

Over the weekend No 10 nonetheless finally realised it had to be seen to do something despite the talk about herd immunity and pushing peaks. With Europe locking down, the worlds banks taking concerted action to prevent a global financial meltdown worse than that of 2008, the news popped up that the government's go-to modellers from Imperial College led by Neil

Ferguson radically changed their forecasts and now predicted that the epidemic curve was on a sharply upwards trajectory. The death tally was by now 35.

Afterwards, some SAGE members slyly defended their own equivocation of the past months by painting a flattering portrait of Cummings's unorthodox attendance of their meetings. He had paid a visit, or visits, despite the Chinese wall between the scientists and the political staff. Supposedly, at this meeting, he was the only one who had the Eureka moment about the virus in contradistinction to all the, presumably myopic, experts Whitehall had managed to select for a seat on the group chaired by Britain's Chief Scientific Adviser or its Chief Medical Officer. Or was it just that everyone knew that Cummings was so vain and convinced of the unique vintage of his mind that he would only believe what was staring them so patently in the face—and Craig Dillon, and Barry Rees, and just about anyone in the country with a job in public health—once the penny finally dropped for him?

13

The Last Stop

The pandemic had reached a critical phase in Britain on 13 March. From single-digit British deaths at the beginning of the week, numbers had ramped up to double digits by the weekend. The number of known infections was close to a thousand. On the plus side, the number of deaths in Italy had reached 492 four days earlier, 97 tallied on the day of the announcement. On that score, the British government still had some time left in its own mind, not least because it looked at Italy with a measure of condescension as a broken nation.

Boris Johnson had finally started chairing COBR meetings and should by now have been fully up to speed. He was at the very least in the same position as Barry Rees in Ceredigion, Professor Friedrich in Groningen and Crown-Prince Salman in Bahrain. In fact, he was in a far better position. Unlike Rees, he could set any budget. Unlike Friedrich, he didn't need to call any friends in Rome, one email by him and a whole department would reach out to their contacts battling in the trenches anywhere in the world. He was even better off than Crown-Prince Salman whose additional budget for the Task Force and War Room and migrant housing improvements was signed off by Bahrain's Prime Minster and the King. As prime minister of the world's sixth largest economy, Johnson could set up a War Chest of half a trillion pounds without much effort against the industrious work of British taxpayers. If money was no object, specialised knowledge was another treasure in limitless supply. With the highest number of Nobel Prize winners after the US, British academics and doctors could crunch any question Johnson might have in a few minutes over the phone.

But Johnson had even more exceptional advantages. Unusual for a British prime minister, if not the first, he had been mayor of one of England's major cities: Britain's biggest city, in fact—London. Like Bahrain, over 40% of its inhabitants were foreign born. For 8 years, Johnson had seen first-hand data how epidemics caused by pathogens were controlled below the level of national government in his city of 9 million inhabitants. On the one hand London had dealt with ongoing bacterial tuberculosis outbreaks as TB capital of Europe, mainly in ethnic communities. Then there was the HIV-virus epidemic. Here new infections also occurred in very specific groups. In 2013, in Johnson's fifth year as mayor, only half of new transmissions occurred among gay men with a median age of 34. There were 45% among heterosexual men and women with a median age of 39 (50% more women than men), the remainder happened among drug users. It equipped, ought to have at any rate, former mayor Johnson with vastly more insight and practical knowledge on the practicalities of epidemics than, say, former biology teacher Barry Rees in Ceredigion.

As London mayor, Johnson had also, for almost a decade, organised central-health support to the local boroughs dealing with the outbreaks of these epidemics in his city.

Here testing had been the game changer in suppressing the epidemics in London's subsets of the population. In fighting the spread of TB there was London's Find & Treat service. The words said it all. The service actively went around London borough hotspots hunting for patients using mobile X-ray scanners rather than wait passively for infectious patients to present themselves at the NHS's A&Es or their GP surgeries. Just waiting for the NHS to deal with London's TB cases, the position to which Dr Harries had announced the cabinet had fallen back to without testing, would have been one sure-fire way of making London's TB crisis unmanageable.

Compared to TB's long history, however, the HIV virus was the novelty pathogen. Even the ancient Egyptians had TB and its diagnosis was well understood, as was the need for intercepting carriers early. But HIV was for decades a lethal, untreatable disease whose infection rate stubbornly refused to be tamed. The explosion of research funding into HIV since the 1980's had subsequently resulted in continuing scientific breakthroughs for HIV and related medical areas. What was known in March 2020 about the coronaviruses, to which COVID-19 belongs, was an off-shoot of that wealth of clinical HIV research, for example.

Johnson understood, then, or should have, that testing is the key to stopping an epidemic by a new virus. During Johnson's mayorship, the big breakthrough was rapid testing. Diagnostic virology, as it is called, was considered expensive until HIV created decades of long-term havoc with medical, social-services and insurance budgets. It was a self-evident truth that pumping money into rapid-testing research would save taxpayer's money all round. In practise, rapid testing meant in London that its health services could start finding HIV carriers through outposts in the affected subsets of its population well before they fell ill and presented themselves to the NHS system.

The rapid HIV tests (the fastest one was 60 seconds) allowed London to suppress the spread of the virus successfully. On World AIDS Day 2013, Johnson had himself emphatically backed the call for more testing. His city, he said, was 'home to almost half the total number of people in the country living with HIV—a fifth of them do not know their status, potentially putting their partners at risk.' There was also a direct research line between the rapid HIV-tests and the research that allowed scientists around the world to put together a test for the virus in a matter of days in January.

Again unusually, Johnson's mindset was also not the ordinary London-centric one for a prime minister. He had led the grass-roots, regional revolt against the EU and what he had painted as Commission diktats—down to its ban of curved bananas, a mythical directive he had written up as the *Telegraph*'s Brussels correspondent early on in his career. More to the point, his government had snatched a decisive victory from Jeremy Corbyn by railroading through Labour's Red Wall in the North of England. He had done so in a manner akin to how he had pulverised London mayor Ken Livingstone by promising the return of double-decker buses. Johnson knew like no other what Whitehall looked like from London or regional England, rather than having a more blinkered view from Kensington or Islington.

So what was he going to do? Now that Whitehall's central community contact-tracing system had gone up in smoke before the epidemic had even started, what ideas did he have up his sleeve?

This was a brilliant opportunity to show off how Britain on its own would outpace its former European counterparts in the EU. All major European countries had stopped large-scale events by 11 March. On 9 March, shambolic Italy even had the temerity to imprison all its citizens inside their own country and houses in a total lockdown, pummelling its economy and precipitating a free fall of its GDP. Only a month earlier, on 3 February, Johnson had waxed disapprovingly about European barriers going up beyond 'what is medically rational to the point of doing real and unnecessary economic damage'. His government was different. He was 'willing at least to make the case powerfully for freedom'. He was 'ready for that role'.

Johnson didn't even have to think like Churchill in war mode and put on his John Bull hat. His own London expertise about the various population subsets and their epidemics was more than enough. One look at the map of Britain and the known COVID outbreaks would have told the prime minister the facts he needed to know and where the virus was entering the UK. The thousand or so confirmed infections were highly localised as in the case of HIV. There was Hampshire and some of the other home counties, South Cumbria, Birmingham and the midlands, and of course London with all its flights coming in and migrant populations. The rest of the country was more or less almost free of the virus at that stage. Their localities pointed at outbreaks within different herds: second homers in Cumbria, returning skiers in the home counties, ethnic minorities in the midlands.

Was he going to keep the majority of the British population unshackled while differentiating the counties that were affected. Was he going to call on his former colleagues in Britain, the mayors and county leaders of the affected areas to discuss with them stringent testing and other methods of containment of the pandemic? Would he ask them what budget they needed and other central support would help in the same way he had dealt with the HIV and TB epidemic in the affected London boroughs? In this way, No 10 would buy time, week by week, to project and organise what it needed to keep deaths and infections at bay and avoid the pitiful sight of Italy with its jumble of makeshift field hospitals for COVID patients.

It would have been daring and require Churchillian dedication. But it would be quite the Brexit masterstroke for freedom. He and Dominic Cummings were later to jump at the opportunity to write a cheque for a 45% investment in the bankrupt Oneweb broadband satellite space venture with an Indian subsidiary belonging to the Mittals. The organisation's workers were largely based in Florida and owed $900 million to Softbank in Japan. Having been turfed out of the European space programme, No 10 must have thought getting in bed on the bounce with a single commercial investor from Asia rather than neighbouring EU nations was a cheap and cheerful answer to the £5 billion cost and rising for a home-spun, sovereign UK system. Championed by business secretary Alok Sharma, signed off by chancellor Rishi Sunak, shot down by mandarin Sam Beckett, No 10 was clearly looking to put its money where its Brexit mouth was, keen to flag up its independence in unusual ways.

Money was clearly no object for another No 10 Brexit-like show of independence from Europe. Going over the heads of Whitehall and coordinating a differentiated approach per local council affected would save the economy, preserve the liberty of the British population who weren't affected, while encircling the virus and containing localised outbreaks. Johnson knew it was a tried and tested approach in local government. Like Barry Rees, he knew that council staff knew exactly what they had to do and only needed to be asked to do it and be given some extra budget to do it right.

Last, but certainly not least, unlike Geoffrey Hacker in Yes Minister, Johnson still had Whitehall tip-toeing around him, desperate to please him as a result of Dominic Cummings' war on mandarins. On 2 January, Cummings had asked for unusual data scientists, software developers, economists, great project managers, junior researchers, communications and policy experts, weirdoes. By now he must surely have found one of each to give Johnson a helping hand in sorting out the details.

As Britain's economy would soar in comparison to the EU, it would teach Whitehall a painful, powerful and instructive lesson about its London-centric, lefty Lacan-toting arrogance. Local councils were not the last remaining pink bits on Whitehall's map of the British Empire. The regions had their own competences and expressed the local power shift that had swept them into office with a resounding majority. Bahrain, Groningen, Ceredigion could do it. Surely Johnson and Cummings were their match? All Britain needed was a leader who gave the freedom of the population the benefit of the doubt, who knew from his own experience how to make it so, like Captain Kirk rather than Superman. And then did it.

Here, then, were the two men who were certain they knew how to square the Brexit hole they had successfully dug. How would they handle the bone that history had thrown them? What would they do with it?

Not a whole lot it turned out.

The Ides of March

It had been a torrid week for Johnson. Beleaguered instead of inspired, Johnson sought to regain control over the facts on the ground and not least the narrative after a week of flipflopping, with the Chief Medical Officer's four-point plan seemingly merging into the Chief Scientific Adviser's *laissez faire* approach. Yet another change in tactic would follow that was to set off a series knockbacks over the next five months. Even then they would yet fight the answer—involve Britain's local governments and their Public Health Directors to go after the disease.

Instead, over the weekend, in waspish words spoken by later-shunned right-wing historian David Starkey, Johnson and Cummings decided 'to fight the Falklands War with a neutron bomb'. The British population would almost instantly start paying the price for their curious mixture of poor thinking, hubris and overreach. The two men set off on a course that would not only ruin Britain's health but also its economy, while creating a raft of problems worse than the COVID epidemic on its own.

On Monday 16 March, Johnson announced daily televised press conferences and said that he was taking 'draconian' measures in limiting the movement of people in Britain. It was to be sure the latest flipflop as only seven days before he had applauded Dr Harries's words that the government 'don't want to disrupt people's lives'.

In his Monday speech he painted yet another picture of his government. There was no billowing cape of liberty. Instead Johnson said, it 'is the time for everyone to stop non-essential contact with others and to stop all unnecessary travel'. The prime minister explained that this included mass gatherings despite what he had said the week before. In a manner that gave the word weaselly a bad name, he added 'we are now moving emphatically away from' them.

If anything Johnson was to supinely copy Europe's lead rather than taking it. 'We need people to start working from home where they possibly can. And you should avoid pubs, clubs, theatres and other such social venues.' Johnson's father Stanley subsequently made clear that he felt free to go to the pub as usual, an indication of Johnson's authority as prime minister.

The former London mayor also addressed the capital directly in a paragraph. Acknowledging implicitly the existence of regional hotspots, he said the city was 'now a few weeks ahead.' But that merited no different approach in itself. Johnson merely repeated, as if in interbellum prime-ministerial homily, what he had said seconds earlier, unless a description of London's pubs and restaurants as 'confined spaces' was meant to convey something of significance Londoners might have missed otherwise.

Was repetition of his own words all the former mayor had come up with as a line of defence for the rest of the country as well those inside, while the city was hit weeks before the rest of the country?

It was particularly odd as that same day he had asked his successor as London Mayor Sadiq Khan to attend the COBR meeting on COVID for the first time. Khan himself had put in several requests as he suspected London would likely be hit hard, without an invitation being extended. Johnson, was in the chair that day, passing questions like a traffic warden to the others in attendance, such as Cummings, senior ministers and civil servants from organisations coordinating the pandemic.

At the meeting Khan was given a document that said that half of Britain's thousand or so known COVID cases were in London. 'I was quite shocked. It was the first time I'd been told this', he told the *Financial Times*. It was extraordinary to think that the mayor had not been given this information before. It was another manifestations of the cabinet's cloak-and-dagger approach to the COVID data in its possession. From that moment, Khan urged Johnson to lock down the capital to encircle the virus in the capital and guard it against breaking out as well as spreading further inside the capital.

It was a portent of Johnson's one-size-fits-all approach, from Westminster down to the rest of the country, that was first to hit the economy like one massive wrecking ball, tearing through British businesses, and then to set off unforeseen cluster bombs as a result of the standstill of economic activity over a four-month period. Hopefully the former classics student had reflected on this.

Two days later and again on Friday, Khan was summoned back to COBR to talk lockdown. 'I was expecting it to be London only', Khan told the *Financial Times*. Johnson was not chairing the meeting on Friday. He was going to give a press conference at 5pm and he was perhaps too busy to attend COBR as well on one and the same day. Michael Gove, Johnson's number five in the cabinet, was in the chair. Those present agreed on basis of Britain's proclivity for partying that the entire country should go in lockdown by the time of Johnson's press conference and so told the prime minster to announce it.

A junior treasury minister, Jesse Norman, however, was also present. He was the only one who dared raise the half-a-trillion pound question. Had there been an analysis of the health impacts of alternatives to a national lockdown and their economic consequences? He was an Etonian with an Oxford classics degree like Johnson, but he had worked at a bank for seven years. The COBR attendees just blanked his question. Like Johnson's absence, it was the elephant in the room. Everyone was just there to dilate on their set of details for the benefit of a decision under Michael Gove's gavel that the absentee prime minister could announce at his press conference.

With the country's key decisions passing only through the minds of just two people—Johnson and Cummings—or really one if rumours are to be believed, there was simply no room to consider what the two weren't interested in or hadn't thought of. They had institutionalised a momentum that had little to do with governing a crisis: Amstrads looking in the mirror, they saw a Fugaku supercomputer. Soon the capacity of both those two minds would be infected and felled by the virus. Yet the institutional momentum would carry on regardless, replicating and enlarging their errors during the make-or-break weeks in the fight against COVID—a butterfly flapping its wings in the Andes. Those temporarily in charge but not in power would wonder, what would No 10 do?

Having disparaged 'experts' during the 2019 general election campaign, in favour of political rhetoric devoid of fact checking, Johnson's government spun round one hundred and eighty degrees, as it saw it was now the time to restore scientists and academics to the frontline, if only to provide a shield for the politicians to hide behind. Once zeros, it was now more convenient to present scientists to the population at large as omniscient priests to the One Truth of fighting COVID with politicians merely nodding respectfully behind them. In response, Britain's academics were to organise their own Independent SAGE on the pandemic to save science from No 10's panto.

Over the weekend of 13 March Professor Neil Ferguson led the charge with a revised epidemiological model that contradicted herd immunity. He now abandoned his scenario 1, the so-called 'mitigation model', in the light of new intelligence from Italy

146

where the health services were under siege. The new model was to be one of 'suppression' or 'flattening the curve' in the hope of delaying the worst of the epidemic to beyond the summer in the hope that good weather may impede the virus and buy some time until treatments or effective vaccines would materialise in time for any winter second wave. Unable to resist flippancy, Boris Johnson termed this 'flattening the sombrero' in another instance of going off-piste. Johnson's 'flattening' measures were to flatten the economy as well. On his watch the UK's worst recession since World War II rationing ended would be announced in August 2020.

This was not the only return to the 1950's, apart from the two thirds of public-school educated minsters—ten times higher than the UK population—in the clubbable government assembled by Johnson. He would later elevate his own brother to the House of Lords in a separate act of cronyism. In public, Johnson and his cabinet would deploy science and civil servants as different coloured pieces of Whitehall plasticine to plug holes in whatever they told Britain about the pandemic. On the day of Johnson's fireside chat with Deputy Chief Medical Officer Dr Harries, for example—would Johnson have had such a knees-together social-media chat with the Chief Medical Officer or Chief Scientific Adviser, or only with one of the seven women of the twenty-six attendees of his cabinet? On that day, Dr Harries said about the use of masks, 'It is usually a bad idea. People tend to leave them on, they contaminate the face mask and then wipe it over something. So it really is not a good idea and it doesn't help'. Scroll forward five months to the day and Johnson would announce on 11 August fines of up to £3200 for failure to wear one in a shop or public transport. Where was the science in all this, other than as Johnson's handmaiden?

Ferguson's model 2's new urgency, if not followed by immediate action certainly, upped the ante and put the National

Health Service in the spotlight. Italy's hospitals had been overwhelmed and had run out of beds, potential shortages of ventilators for intensive care loomed large, as would later oxygen supplies. Health minister Matt Hancock was left to organise the effort. With a note of desperation he invited carmakers and defence contractors to switch production to make ventilators, calling on the Unipart Group, among others to put themselves on a war footing, as a national priority.

Johnson himself needed no further prompting to embark on a round of Second World War rhetoric, inflating it to that of Winston Churchill. It was far easier to posture as a latter-day Churchill while throttling liberty than to do the hard work. In June, Johnson would go for more government-by-posturing as he assumed the mantle of another well-known leader in Western history—Franklin D. Roosevelt. Westminster would aid and abet in putting up such *tableaux vivants* like staff in a nineteenth-century country house. Statistical projections would be shown like releases of doves never to be seen again. Leaving at the close of the London season like a land-owning gent, Johnson would disappear to an inaccessible part of Scotland for July holidays in a media void. For a government that prided itself on being in tune with the public mood, it was another shot in the foot. Regaining the narrative in the face of the leitmotif of doing too little too late, being too hands-off, too lazy, too self-satisfied and too patrician, became an uphill battle as real facts piled up against never-ending spin.

Around the country the public, becoming impatient, increasingly uncertain about what was going on, had already started to withdraw into the sanctuary of their own homes and avoid meetings, to call for school closures and to organise themselves into an estimated 720 citizens armies to look after the most vulnerable in society by volunteering to pick up shopping, deliver medicine and even to deliver music lessons to relieve boredom.

With its London-centric and NHS focus it would be some weeks before the government would cotton on to the importance of public engagement and then in a cack-handed top-down way the NHS would muster a volunteer force of 750,000 people without knowing what to do with them. Unlike Professor Friedrich's Groningen volunteers, this standing army of good citizens would wait and wait to be put to useful work. From China to Bahrain and Bahrain to Cuba the social mobilisation of volunteers became a key factor in contact tracing and keeping people safe by monitoring the comings and goings of everyday life, combining the low tech use of home visits and temperature screening at the doors of schools and supermarkets with the high tech application of wrist bands and dedicated phone Apps to identify risky social encounters. Not so in Britain, leaving sombrero jokes to one side.

On Thursday, 19 March just one week after the government had abandoned community testing, Johnson announced an ambition to increase testing to 25,000 a day from the current level of 4,000. This compared with the existing German level of 12,000 a day. Whilst local general practitioners and Directors of Public Health remained on the sidelines, unable to test those with symptoms or get a handle on the spread of the virus in their local communities, celebrities, sports stars, the wealthy and business people were paying £295 to private clinics for tests that offered results in 72 hours.

That same day the false promise surfaced of an antibody test to identify those who had already been infected and might be presumed to be able to work unhindered. The prime minister announced that 'we are close to a test that reveals who is immune'. This red herring would continue to distract attention from the dire state of testing capacity in the months ahead as would over-optimist claims for the rapid development of a vaccine to stop the virus in its tracks; something that had eluded scientists with SARS,

149

Swine 'flu and Ebola before. Three days later the army would seize the testing equipment to be found in university laboratories around the country. It was subsequently unclear what happened to it with a resonance to the melting down of railings and kitchen pots and pans at the height of World War II.

Boris Johnson's announcement was the first shot in a battle to control the narrative about preparedness and capacity that extended to ventilators, oxygen and Personal Protective Equipment (PPE) that would run and run. The related issue of face masks and face coverings would become one which brought the issues of the evidence base and the political imperatives into sharp focus.

As more knowledge accumulated about the new coronavirus, so did understanding about its infectivity. Thousands of coronaviruses exist with four of them being responsible for many common colds and two responsible for SARS and MERS. Whereas those infected with SARS did not transmit it until 24-36 hours after displaying symptoms and people could be isolated before they could spread it to others, new scientific data suggested that people with COVID-19 could transmit the virus before they showed definite symptoms. In addition, as a droplet-and-aerosol borne virus it can be readily spread when a carrier coughs or exhales and can be caught from inhalation or touching the eyes, nose or mouth with hands that have been in contact with the virus. It could, in addition, survive for up to 36 hours on hard surfaces such as kitchen work surfaces, light switches, door and lavatory handles. Rigorous personal and environmental hygiene was the first line of defence, together with reducing levels of social contact and mixing and for those in frontline clinical and regular face-to-face situations with those potentially infected, as well as PPE was essential.

The issue of PPE first came to general public attention during the Ebola epidemic of 2014 in West Africa. Here was a highly contagious viral disease, spread by close personal and intimate contact, particularly infecting frontline clinical workers and relatives of the deceased involved with ritual washing of the body, bringing with it a case mortality rate of around 50%. Great efforts were made to train up local staff and international volunteers in wearing elaborate Hazmat clothing to protect them from the Ebola virus.

One might have thought that one of the lessons of this outbreak would have been that adequate supplies of PPE should be held in store as part of resilient preparedness for health emergencies. That this was the case was one of the messages from Operation Cygnus in 2016 which revealed that faced with a pandemic of influenza there was not sufficient PPE to go round, never mind the shortage of ventilators and mortuary capacity.

Despite building public pressure to publish the Cygnus report it only saw the light of day when it was leaked to the *Guardian*, who would publish its main findings on May 7. Earlier, on April 27, a BBC Panorama programme caused a major controversy when it revealed that such stocks of PPE as had been held in store had been allowed to go past their 'use by' date and had had their date stamps repeatedly changed.

Another announcement that would have lethal consequences followed. The same programme revealed that on the same day that Boris Johnson had expressed his ambition for 25,000 tests a day and trailed both an antibody test and the advent of a vaccine, the new COVID virus, which had initially been classified as being in the highest category of infectious disease, was being re-designated to a lower category of risk.

In January, when the new coronavirus was first identified it had been classified internationally as being able to cause a 'High Consequence Infectious Disease' or HCID. However on March 19, with hospital admissions escalating and the shortage of PPE becoming ever more apparent, it was re-designated to a lower category of risk known as 'Hazgroup3', or HG3, following a meeting of Britain's Four Nations Group together with the Advisory Committee on Dangerous Pathogens.

The criteria for classifying a pathogen as an HCID were very specific. They included an organism that produced an illness that was: acute; had a high-case fatality rate; there was no effective treatment nor specific preventive intervention; it was difficult to recognise quickly; it could spread in the health care system; and it required an enhanced systematic response in order to deal effectively with it. On the face of it, COVID-19 met each of these criteria but the justification for reclassifying it was given on the grounds that the mortality rate at that time was believed to be 0.6% (which was still greater than seasonal 'flu), and that there was now the potential to identify and control it through testing. In retrospect this may have been true if the UK had been following WHO advice.

The consequences of downgrading the virus to HG3 were that it made it possible to conform to existing protocols. Patients could be treated in non-specialist hospital beds that did not conform to the rigorous standards in infectious disease units. It also meant that the safety specification for PPE for staff caring for COVID-19 patients could be revised downwards. In the days and weeks ahead the consequences would be severe, in terms of within-hospital spread of the virus, the spread of the virus to care homes and out into the community and the unnecessary deaths of many including hundreds of doctors, nurses and other frontline staff in the NHS.

Later, on 11 June, Rajeev Syal, in the *Guardian*, would report damming National Audit Office findings that the government had failed to stockpile gowns and visors despite warnings to do so and that less than half the expected pieces of certain equipment were handed out to frontline workers as the crisis developed. The only categories of PPE of which stocks had been increased following the emerging news from China, in January, had been aprons and clinical waste bags. It was also revealed that NERVTAG, the New and Emerging Virus Threats Advisory Group, had recommended in June 2019 that PHE should stockpile gowns and switch from glasses to visors when glasses were being restocked.

One of the major weaknesses in the supply chain and stockpiling of PPE for major emergencies was the dependence on just-in-time supply, which had been widely adopted in the NHS from private sector practice over the previous twenty five years as a device to avoid tying up large financial commitments in stock. This had been revealed during the 2000 fuel protests that had brought the country to a standstill and created a major political crisis for the Blair government, not least because of its impact on continuity of NHS care at the time. Nobody seems to have learned the lesson then or since.

In February it was reported that PHE had stocks of 83 million gloves (41.5 million pairs), 25.7 million pairs of eye protectors and 156 million face masks, but by the end of April none were left. The news that various announcements of large numbers of PPE items being procured in government press conferences was double counting, for example each glove constituting one item, caused outrage when it was revealed in the Panorama programme on April 27. The use of large hypothetical numbers in itself and devoid of context, was a recurring theme of the cabinet's 'numbers game' played out regularly in the daily press conferences; for example with no information about the large numbers of full personal protection kit that each frontline worker needed for biosecurity in the course of a shift.

In the desperate search for PPE supplies the government first turned to the big brand names such as Barbour and Burberry, presumably best known to members of the Johnson cabinet and the special advisers under Cummings's control from No 10. Whitehall could only conceive of a few large suppliers producing the quantities that were required. Yet there were myriads of small-and-medium business suppliers in Britain, including the owners of still functioning textile mills in Lancashire, who could produce the shortfall but weren't given orders. When corporate sources were slow to deliver, a much heralded consignment of 400,000 surgical gowns was announced from Turkey on 22 April. It finally arrived two days late with only 10% of the order, which failed to meet the specification and was rejected, a similar fate had already met testing kits from China

The pattern of overpromising and underdelivering was becoming a character trait of the UK response. It was to have a particular impact on the residents and staff of care homes, for whom PPE was to be a long time coming. They were to pay the price in increased infections. Former Health Secretary and now Chair of the Health Select Committee, Jeremy Hunt, would later be quoted as saying 'it seems extraordinary that no-one appeared to consider the clinical risk to care homes, despite widespread knowledge that the virus could be spread asymptomatically'.

The political storm that followed the Panorama programme on April 27 would mark the beginning of the wider politicisation of the crisis with allegations by allies of the government of political bias against the BBC and a succession of attempts to discredit commentators who criticised the government's handling of the emergency.

Ventilators, Oxygen and Beds

When it came to ventilators the UK was again caught flat footed, having failed to heed either its own historic Influenza Pandemic Planning Guidance or the lessons from the Cygnus exercise in 2016. Both had shown that in the event of a major respiratory epidemic emergency many more ventilators and intensive care beds would be needed. This situation had been compounded in February when the UK government had failed to join in the consortium of European Union countries in securing adequate supplies for testing, personal protection and for ventilators. Whether because of a post-Brexit mentality or a breakdown of communications was contested but the consequences were severe.

Once the numbers of severely ill patients had begun to climb health secretary Matt Hancock's response had been to challenge the British engineering industry to divert their production lines to meet the challenge. On March 20 he was reported in *The Times* as saying 'if you produce a ventilator we will buy it. No number is too high', his department indicating that in a worst case scenario another 20,000 would be needed and that funding from the foreign aid budget was to be diverted to produce ventilators for the UK. Under the umbrella of a consortium 'Ventilator Challenge' more than a dozen companies from the aviation and automotive industries had joined the consortium including, Siemens, Airbus, engineers from the Formula One teams, Rolls Royce and Dyson. James Dyson appeared to jump the gun when he claimed to have a contract for 10,000 machines for the NHS.

While this work was going on clinical understanding of the pathology caused by the virus was developing and it would later become clear that far from being primarily a respiratory/pulmonary disease, the clinical picture extended to range of organ system involvement that could include the brain, kidneys and liver with serious thromboembolic impact and that many of those who were put on incubators would die. As clinical practice evolved only half of the sickest patients came to have deep invasive ventilation with the alternative of Continuous Positive Airways Pressure (Cpap), demonstrating better outcomes.

Writing in the *Guardian* on 26 April Sarah Boseley put it that, 'the rush to increase the number of ventilators in Britain from 8,000 to 18,000 was a response to an early assumption that intubation was the only way to save lives of those who became severely ill. Industry was urged to switch production and Dyson was among the companies volunteering to help, but it has now been told by the government that its services are not needed'. By 7 May it looked as though most of the additional capacity would be surplus to requirements, another example of doing too much too late.

Hospitals, beds and oxygen

As the epidemic in Italy had risen to a crescendo earlier in March hospitals, had been overwhelmed with patients with insufficient intensive care capacity and ventilators and oxygen to supply them. Somewhere between two and four weeks behind Italy, reflecting the incubation period of those returning to the UK from half-term skiing, the window of opportunity to do some catching up was small. The belated recognition of the urgency was causing a frantic rearranging of life lifeboats as the iceberg drew closer.

Of prime political importance was seen to be the resilience of the NHS hospitals and their beds in the face of the rising tide of admissions, something that would lead to the creation of a vast new hospital facility in the Exel conference centre in short order and to the early discharge of large numbers of hospital patients to their homes and to care homes. The NHS Executive and NHS Improvement direction was' to release all patients medically fit to leave' to free up bed space.

The *Health Service Journal* would report on 5 April that several NHS Trusts in London would get engineering support to increase oxygen supplies amid concerns that hospitals were running short of hospital gases as a result of the high levels of demand on the piped hospital systems. Some hospitals were drawing off more oxygen through the pipes than the systems were designed for. Concern was expressed that it might be necessary to supplement these piped supplies with bedside oxygen cylinders, compromising the supply to patients with Chronic Obstructive Airways Disease in the community, who depended on cylinder supplies. At this point in early April, with one week to go before the predicted peak of the epidemic curve, oxygen supply issues had been reported from multiple hospitals.

While the country was being prepared for the worst days of the emergency in a mood of increasing alarm, with panic buying still occurring in the shops, and concerns being expressed about people's willingness to adhere to voluntary spacing, physicians were collaborating internationally to try and find optimal treatment regimes for sick patients. Word from China had supported the use of a cocktail of medicines that included the anti-retro viral drugs that had been used in the treatment of HIV and Ebola, together with antibiotics and the antimalarial hydroxy-chloroquine. Chinese researchers had claimed benefit from both hydroxychloroquine and the anti-viral, remdesivir and a study from France had claimed that 70% of 36 patients treated with hydroxy-chloroquine got rid of the virus in 3-6 days.

NHS clinicians were extremely sceptical about the claims for the highly toxic hydroxychloroquine, despite enormous political and commercial pressure to adopt its use not least from American President Trump. They preferred to wait for the results of properly constructed trials. This would become a subplot that caught up the *Lancet* in the publication of a paper claiming to show no effect of hydroxychloroquine that was subsequently discredited whilst evidence emerged of some benefit from remdesivir and significant benefit from an old established preparation dexametha-sone, a steroid with inflammatory suppression qualities.

A National State of Emergency
These considerations must have been very much in mind when the prime minister addressed the nation on Monday March 23 amid mounting alarm and declared a national state of emergency. Announcing the greatest restriction in individual liberty in history, Johnson introduced a complete lockdown to come into operation

on Thursday 26 March. People were banned from leaving their homes or meeting in groups of more than two, and to maintain a distance of two metres from each other, something that would be translated swiftly into a British version of two yards.

Thirteen days later, on 5 April, the Queen addressed the nation to an audience of 24 million, only the fifth time she had made such an address in her 68 years as monarch. Capturing the popular mood she struck a positive tone in claiming that the UK 'will succeed' in its fight against coronavirus, paid tribute to key workers and thanked people for following the rules to stay indoors, before quoting Vera Lynn's wartime rallying song lyrics 'we'll meet again'.

Throughout March the numbers of reported hospital deaths increased sharply from 144 on Thursday 19, the day that Boris Johnson spoke of his target for testing of 25,000 a day, to 442 on March 24, when he declared a National State of Emergency and again to 621 on April 5 when the Queen addressed the nation. During this time the shortage of PPE took off as a focus of concern and of the media.

The wealthy had been reported as fleeing to their second homes in the country; plans had been mooted to turn hotels into hospitals to increase capacity; whilst modellers were predicting 20-25% sickness and self-isolating absence by healthcare staff, doctors had wrongly been told to continue working even if family members were infected; soldiers had been put on standby to deliver oxygen supplies; online supermarket order lines were crashing; chancellor Rishi Sunak had announced an 'unprecedented financial package to protect the economy or unprecedented times'; there had been outbreaks of COVID-19 associated with the gatherings of the religiously devout; private cardiologist Dr Mark Ali was reported as having taken £2.5 m from carrying out private COVID-19 tests in his Harley Street practice; GPs had written letters to over 2 million especially vulnerable patients telling them to shield themselves at home; legislation had been passed to make it easier to section those with mental health problems. By now the nations' schools had been shut down and the GCSE and 'A' level exams cancelled for the first time in their history.

Meanwhile the *Sunday Times* reported that behind the scenes in Whitehall Dominic Raab, Michael Gove, Rishi Sunak and Matt Hancock were jostling to take charge should Boris Johnson fall ill.

14

Politically-Led Science and the Numbers Game

The Whitehall Rock

Public health is concerned with understanding the causes of ill health in the places where people live out their lives, and taking action to prevent it and to protect the population. From the 1840's onwards, when Bismarck introduced social reforms in Germany, faced with rapid urbanisation, insurrection and the threat of revolution, most progressive states came to accept that responsibility for public health lay with government. At that time the argument between those who saw the role of government as being solely to protect people's property and those who argued that as the only property most people had was their health, it was a primary government responsibility to protect their citizens against disease as much as defence against foreign aggression and domestic instability, seemed to have been resolved.

Charles Winslow, the first Dean of the Yale School of Public Health, captured the scope of the enterprise in his 1920's definition that has proved enduring: 'Public health is the science and art of preventing disease, prolonging life and promoting physical health and efficiency through organised community efforts for the sanitation of the environment, the education of the individual in principles of personal hygiene, the organisation of medical and nursing service for the early diagnosis and preventive treatment of disease, and the development of the social machinery which will ensure to every individual in the community a standard of living adequate for the maintenance of health'.

This reasoning was very much in line with that of the famous cell biologist, Rudolf Virchov, for whom 'Medicine is a social science and politics is nothing more than medicine on a large scale'. Others have argued that 'public health is the political wing of medicine' and that 'parliament is the dispensary of public health'.

That the 'art and science' of public health is intimately entangled with political decisions has long been at the heart of training for the practice of public health in the UK. Nevertheless tensions periodically surface between the worlds of the researcher or the personal clinician and that of the public-health practitioner, and the need to square the circle of Geoffrey Rose's requirement that the practice of public health requires 'a clean mind and dirty hands'. The close, challenging, often difficult, yet respectful and mutually supportive nature of effective relationships between senior politicians and their public-health advisers, that makes for sound policy making and intervention, is explored in Sally Sheard and Liam Donaldson's history of the role of the Chief Medical Officer, *The Nation's Doctor*.

In recent years the chaotic changes of the arrangements for public health in England, together with the revival of free market ideology internationally, has threatened the longstanding consensus of the role of public health. The naive belief that public health is a cost rather than an investment in economic and social development has come to threaten both.

The politics of COVID-19
Public health in England was not in good shape when COVID-19 arrived from China at the end of January 2020. Neglect of the system and of health emergency planning combined with political

161

dysfunction arising from over three years of obsession with Brexit. One catastrophic result was that the impending external epidemic threat did not receive the attention that was needed. Of crucial importance, was that a new prime minister and a new Chief Medical Officer had yet to develop that challenging, yet supportive relationship that would be so essential if the public health was to be effective and not put in jeopardy. The third person who would figure prominently as one of the public faces and principal actors of the COVID emergency was to be the Chief Scientific Adviser, Sir Patrick Vallance.

By now Boris Johnson's persona and modus operandi were a public secret. Widely regarded as someone who was more interested in winning elections than in following through with delivery, he resembled Baron von Munchhausen, with his fantastical dreams, rather than a grounded leader with a plan. He had a track record of wild and off-the-cuff schemes that made headlines but never came to anything or that left messes behind for others to clear up: second hand water cannons from Germany that went unused and a garden bridge that cost millions but was unviable and later as prime minister, as COVID-19 spread, an attention-distracting fantasy bridge linking Northern Ireland to Scotland. Subsequently, both before and after falling sick with the virus, he was rapidly seen as the invisible leader.

The new Chief Medical Officer, Professor Chris Whitty had taken up his post, succeeding Dame Sally Davies, in October 2019, having previously had a career as an academic clinical epidemiologist, practising medicine in infectious diseases at University College hospital. He had experience of working on research into Ebola in Sierra Leone with lead statistical modeller, Professor Neil Ferguson from Imperial College and Sir Jeremy Farrar, the Director of the Wellcome Trust, both of whom would be members of the government committee, SAGE, which would advise on the management of the COVID-19 pandemic in the UK.

Chris Whitty's epidemiological background appears to have consisted of the one-year MSc in Epidemiology at the London School of Hygiene and Tropical Medicine rather than the more comprehensive, Masters in Public Health degree as part of a five year post-graduate training in public health, which was seen as an essential prerequisite for comprehensive training in the practical aspects of the discipline. His membership of the Faculty of Public Health was a bestowed honour, rather than one attained by examination.

Although highly regarded by his colleagues as an intelligent, dependable but very private man, in contrast to the prime minister, Whitty came very much from the academic tradition of clinical epidemiology, rather than the practical route of grass roots and local public-health practice. This was something that was to become a general issue in terms of all those called on to advise government through SAGE. There was both a lack of shoe-leather and practical public-health consultants, as well as the pre-dominance of clubbable academics from tight London and Oxbridge, social, academic, and chum bubbles.

The third of the triumvirate, Sir Patrick Vallance, was also a physician and scientist with a background in cell physiology, clinical pharmacology and the pharmacological industry—where he had been head of research and development at Glaxo Smith Kline—but not in public health. At Glaxo his contribution had met with mixed reviews. He had also played a controversial role in the aftermath of the Grenfell Tower fire tragedy, chairing the Scientific Advisory Group (SAG), for the review of potential environmental contamination in Grenfell and North Kensington. It was a group that also included Chris Whitty. Later he was to be on the panel that appointed Whitty to the post of Chief Medical Officer.

Criticism of the handling of the public-health aftermath by the Royal Borough of Kensington and Chelsea centred on why tests on soil and residues for toxic products of combustion had not been carried out immediately after the fire. A lack of both environmental and public-health capacity in the borough council, to carry out appropriate tests had been a key factor, but so too had been the advice by Public Health England's then Regional Director of Public Health for London, Yvonne Doyle, that such testing was unnecessary. Later, in response to a public outcry from the survivors and bereaved, and affected local residents of the Grenfell fire, Sir Patrick's SAG had assumed responsibility but was also criticised for not listening to the concerns of those affected and failing to carry through the testing deemed necessary by outside experts.

In her resignation letter from the SAG in August 2019, independent combustion toxicologist consultant Professor Anna Stec said that 'nothing is in place to assess environmental and health risks', initial research having found that toxicity of dust and debris around the tower, where 71 people had died, was 160 times higher in the North Kensington area than normal. In her letter to Sir Patrick, Professor Stec said that, 'there are still a significant number of people suffering physically and mentally following the Grenfell Tower fire, and yet, there is still nothing in place to properly evaluate all the adverse health effects of the fire, and specifically exposure to fire effluents'.

When it came to COVID-19 and SAGE the omens were not looking good.

Leadership and communications
Official guidance, as well as experience from previous major public-health emergencies, teaches us that openness and transparency, together with readily identifiable and trusted voices, are essential if the public is to be kept onboard. This is especially the case if social mobilisation becomes necessary and tough decisions affecting people's lives taken. From the first returning travellers

from Wuhan, who had been quarantined at Arrowe Park without prior public warning, there were suggestions that this may become a problem.

Ideally consistent authoritative professional and recognisable figures are needed at national and regional and local levels, standing alongside, and supporting, but clearly independent of, political leaders. With the government boycott of the BBC and the late appearance of the Chief Medical Officer at the national level the opportunity to take the necessary initiative was missed, leading later to an ongoing fight to control the narrative.

The gagging by PHE and by local authorities of local Directors of Public Health was an own goal. In the absence of coherent and trusted voices rumours began to spread about the nature of the virus and the infection, together with quack cures. National and local print and media journalists reported that they were unable to obtain interviews with senior spokespeople from the NHS, the Department of Health or Public Health England, which was particularly inclined to be invisible throughout the emergency. It would be a long time before there was any systematic rebuttal of 'fake news' as had been done from the early days in Bahrain with its commitment to open public engagement. Matters were not helped by the lack of public information about what had happened to those quarantined from Wuhan after their 14 days in isolation, the withholding of information about those testing positive for the virus and the increasingly obvious disinterest of the prime minister in anything other than family matters or Brexit.

In the early weeks of the emergency, the government standing in the opinion polls held up, but public confidence began to wane, especially following the distressing sequence of events in the week of 9 March when, with the reported numbers of those infected and hospital deaths doubling every two to three days, there was rapidly increasing public disquiet over large scale events taking place. The government plan, such as it was, based on the Johnson-Whitty four stages was beginning to give way to Johnson's notion of 'squash the sombrero'. The fiasco over herd immunity and the subsequent u-turn and mixed messages on the epidemic trajectory from Imperial College modellers lay behind Boris Johnson's attempts to shore up public confidence and respond to criticism of No 10 for lack of transparency by introducing the first press conference from 10 Downing Street on Monday 16 March.

Press-conference symbolism

The first press conference set the tone for what were to become mostly daily events for the next three months, initially with the prime minister flanked on either side by the Chief Medical Officer and the government's Chief Scientific Adviser, Patrick Vallance. Each of these three principal figures stood at a podium against a backdrop of two union flags; this nationalistic tone being reinforced in future conferences by frequent references to World War II.

The new mantra, adding to the public invocation to 'wash your hands' was that the government would be 'following the science', something that would later come to be highly contested. The presence of a gallery of reporters from the media, together with the three spokespeople in a relatively crowded room, was in contrast to the emerging message about social distancing, an example of cognitive dissonance that would later backfire spectacularly when a number of those involved tested positive for the virus.

It was announced that these conferences would normally be led by the prime minister or senior ministers and their senior advisers. In reality there came to be a constantly changing cast of characters with quite regular appearances by health secretary Matt Hancock, solid NHS Medical Director, Stephen Powis, and the

Chief Scientific Adviser, whose interventions over herd immunity and assertion that less than 20,000 deaths would be a good result, would come to define a sense of complacency. Less regular appearances were made by the Chief Medical Officer who was frequently deputised for by Deputy Chief Medical Officer Jennie Harries, whose contributions would often raise questions among public-health colleagues, and less frequently by Deputy Chief Medical Officer Jonathan Van-Tam, who was to reveal a welcome streak of integrity following the Dominic Cummings breach of lockdown in late May.

The prime minister in keeping with his invisibility record made the least appearances of the principal actors. Later, as the financial aspects of the crisis loomed large, chancellor, Rishi Sunak became a prominent attendee promising that he would do 'whatever it takes' to deal with the emergency. It was to prove no more imaginative than writing large cheques drawn on half a trillion pounds of borrowed money in the hope that they would plug the hole Johnson had struck at the heart of the economy.

In addition to these politicians and advisers there was a steady flow of ministers from other government departments, including the ambitious Michael Gove from the Cabinet Office, accident prone Grant Shapps from Transport, recurrent liability Priti Patel from the Home Office, and lightweight Helen Whateley from Health and Social Care.

The input from Public Health England was intermittent and confused, the agency itself being largely invisible in most stages of the emergency with little sign of Chief Executive, Duncan Selbie. Yvonne Doyle, who had been promoted to PHE Medical Director, in 2019 from her role as Director of Public Health for London, where her public appearances had been heavily criticised by the Grenfell campaigners, was not much in evidence at first but later made intermittent showings as did her predecessor Paul Cosford, who had taken early retirement on ill-health grounds over a year before. John Newton, PHE's Chief Knowledge Officer, was brought in with fanfare to head up the governments antibody testing initiative in April but disappeared from sight once the value of this became unclear.

The format for the press conferences initially involved an introduction by the politician or one of his colleagues, that included any new measures that were to be taken, followed by one of the government advisers being brought in to make a slide presentation of the current state of play with regard to numbers of those testing positive in the previous 24 hours, hospital admissions and impact on hospital beds, and finally the number of new deaths. Following the national lockdown on 26 March there was also included a slide showing national transport flows as a proxy measure for its impact on peoples movements. Finally there was a question and answer session with invited journalists.

The government and its advisers were still struggling and even the mild natured Chief Medical Officer was becoming rattled, being reported in the *Irish Times* of March 21 as having 'complained on Thursday about "ranting" critics of the British approach, adding that testing and containment was no longer a viable strategy'. It was only the beginning of the crisis for Professor Whitty.

Within a week, and with lockdown now in place, it became clear that the one thing that was running very smoothly indeed was a new approach to communications to act as a Chinese wall to hold the fort against the gathering pace of the pandemic's bad news on the ground. The cabinet's public relations were to be run like a political campaign. On March 29, Boris Johnson drafted in a new team of communications advisers headed up by a protege of Lynton Crosby, Isaac Levido, who had run the Johnson general election campaign in 2019. Levido would work closely with Dominic Cummings.

Having already adopted a political campaign 'grid' of communications for the daily press conferences the intention was to sharpen up the messages epitomised by a further mantra, to be repeated regularly of 'Stay Home, Protect the NHS, Save Lives'. The provenance of this was clearly in line with 'Get Brexit Done' and 'Take Back Control', which had worked so well for the general election campaign. The clear intention was to restore the prime minister's reputation for competence and regain control of the narrative. How this would fit with openness and transparency, with 'following the science' and with evidence-based public health was another issue.

As the reported daily death toll grew from 209 on 29 March to 621 a week later, when the Queen spoke to the nation, the core narrative that the government wished to put in place continued to emphasise that 'it was following the science'. Questions about testing and tracing and about PPE were met with increasingly extravagant claims about what was possible, what was happening, and why the UK with the best scientists and the best public health had no need to follow the practices from other countries even though they may be showing more success. In the weeks ahead it would become ever more apparent that the press conferences were heavily stage managed with vetting of those journalists being admitted and preselection of their questions, which were rarely answered frankly especially if they proved penetrating.

Channel 4 television, the BBC and journalists from scientific publications were among those who had particular difficulty in obtaining invitations. There was an increasing sense that the professional position and integrity of the government's advisers was being placed in jeopardy in such politically stage managed events and that their positioning alongside the prime minister or his deputy was implying co-option into politics rather than science. Ironically, those who questioned the validity of the approach and asking for transparency of the evidence that decisions were being taken by the government, its advisers and agencies, began to be accused of being politically motivated. Increasingly they were subject to personal attacks involving 'bots' on social media together with efforts to have them excluded from mainstream medium, especially the BBC, on the grounds that they had political motives or that they harboured darker prejudices.

There were lots of questions beginning to be asked, not just by reporters but by the general public across the country. There was increasing frustration that questions were not being fully answered or avoided altogether, and questions began to be asked about the advice that the government and its advisers was getting and where it was coming from.

This had begun on the weekend of 14 March when Imperial College modeller Neil Ferguson had never been out of the headlines during the row over herd immunity. His admission that the projections for the epidemic curve that advisors had been working with had been flawed had led to the dramatic change of policy direction by the government.

Leader of one of three principle modelling groups from Imperial College, the London School of Hygiene and Tropical Medicine and Oxford University, Ferguson had been held up as one of the world's great modellers despite his techniques having been previously criticised by vets and farmers for having led to the unnecessary slaughter of millions of cattle and sheep in the foot and mouth epidemic in 2001. Around the country, less lauded practitioners, academics and amateurs had been looking at the daily reported numbers and calculating on the back of envelopes or on pocket calculators where things were heading, mostly concluding that they were out of control and that unless something drastic was done the country was looking at tens if not hundreds of thousands of deaths in the near future.

Nowhere was the confusion and concern more than with the succession of numbers that filled the press conference sessions: the size of the testing capacity for COVID-19, who had access to them, the numbers of tests actually done, and done satisfactorily; the results of tests and their validity; the amounts of available PPE and who had access to it; the numbers of new cases of COVID, hospital admissions and deaths. There was confusion about the relative potential contribution of antigen and antibody testing and whether antibody testing had any value at all; wild optimism was generated about the prospects for vaccine development and for treatment options, only for these to be dashed by cold reality.

The person who frames the question determines the range of solutions. In this case the public was being asked to trust the numbers, to trust the basis of the advice the government was getting and to trust the actions that it was taking. The public was being kept in the dark and increasingly feeling patronised by leaders who were in plain sight. At which point many of these omniscient people began to go down with COVID-19.

The first member of the government and its advisers to have been reported as self-isolating with coronavirus had been mental-health minister Nadine Dorries on March 7. Now she was to be followed by a flurry of others beginning with Matt Hancock, Chris Whitty and Duncan Selbie on March 26. According to the *Health Service Journal*, Selbie was continuing to lead PHE's response to the coronavirus crisis from home. Prince Charles reported sick the same day, followed by prime minister Boris Johnson on 4 and Michael Gove on 7 April. It seemed as if the country's leaders had been following the age old advice to 'do as I say not what I do'. The prime minister's reckless behaviour in shaking hands with 'everybody' on a hospital visit had put himself at risk and brought to a head the question of who would deputise for him as leader of the country—the answer, Dominic Raab. As Johnson's health deteriorated over the next two days and he was admitted to hospital and intensive care, heralding another month long absence, the numbers game was becoming more and more fraught as it became clear that rather than following the science, the science was following the politics.

R0, the reproduction number of COVID-19

With lockdown in place from 26 March and the numbers of deaths climbing towards its peak in early April, the public became familiar with the concept of Ro, or the reproduction number. In an epidemic situation the critical factor is how many cases are generated from each person who is ill and infects others, if this is greater than 1.0 the infection will spread, potentially exponentially. If the R0 is less than 1.0 it will spread slowly and eventually die out. The R0 is affected by such factors as the infectivity of the organism, the numbers of people in a population who have no resistance to it and are susceptible to infection, the population density and the rate of disappearance of the virus from the population by recovery or death of those affected. R0 itself refers to the situation at the beginning of an outbreak when there may be no or little resistance to the infection among the population and differs from the later situation when some or many people may have developed resistance and the effective reproduction number (Re) will be less.

This became an important issue during the COVID pandemic because of the confusing misuse of these terms, not least in the press conferences where the 'R' being quoted was an average based on the availability of test results. In reality different 'R' numbers were to be found in different areas, groups and settings across the country depending on what stage they were on their own epidemic curves. In practical terms COVID-19 was seeded at different times in different places, probably beginning in areas where people had returned from skiing in Italy and Austria with early clusters being seen in some of the better off parts of the country, followed by clusters relating to specific seeding events such as the mass gatherings in Bristol, Cheltenham and Liverpool, as well as among some congregating faith communities. Later the outbreaks in care homes and prisons would begin to run their courses as separate phenomena and the epidemic would spread across the country gathering momentum especially among poorer and black and minority ethnic (BAME) communities.

The situation in early April in the UK was that with a doubling of the numbers of cases and deaths every two to three days the overall R0 appeared to be in the range of 2.0-4.0. The lockdown was hoped to reduce this to below 1.0 and regain control of the situation that had been allowed to develop.

The real numbers of COVID deaths
In mid-March, as the number of confirmed cases had risen by 407 in 24 hrs to 1,950, the government's Chief Scientific Adviser told the Health Select Committee that keeping the coronavirus death toll below 20,000 would be a good result. He went on to make a comparison with an annual total of excess deaths from winter 'flu of about 8,000. Within a short time the whole basis of these numbers would be thrown into doubt as it became clear that the only cases and deaths that were being counted were those where a clinical diagnosis, usually in hospital, had been confirmed by a test. Cases and deaths outside hospitals, either at home, in care homes, prisons or elsewhere were politically conveniently out of sight and out of mind. This state of affairs was to continue in one way and another for months to come with 'butter wouldn't melt in their mouths' statements of cases and death numbers from ministers and their advisers in the daily press conferences.

On 31 March the *Guardian* reported that in response to the criticism of the published figures from the NHS and Public Health England, the Office of National Statistics would in future begin to publish regular figures for all deaths, including those occurring outside hospitals, where COVID-19 was a suspected cause. The explanation given for the previous incompleteness of the data was the time taken for the paperwork to pass through the coroner's office. The spotlight having been thrown on this issue it soon became clear that even this more complete set of statistics would still be a significant underestimate of the numbers of COVID deaths in the absence of extensive testing in both care homes and other community settings including the home.

A welcome intervention by James Tozer of the *Economist* magazine began to throw light on the significant shortfall in the numbers of deaths being reported, not least in the emerging catastrophe in the nations care homes which eventually accounted for probably around half of all deaths. It would also emerge later that dozens, if not hundreds of people had died alone, at home from what may have been COVID. Eventually most apolitical observers came to accept that the most reliable estimate of the numbers of COVID deaths was to be derived from a comparison of the all causes excess deaths during the epidemic with the average for the previous five years, a calculation that added about 50% to the figures that the government continued to publish. Even then it seemed that manipulation of the totals was routinely taking place.

If the government had been keen to keep the total number of published deaths below the Chief Scientific Adviser's idea of a 'good result' at 20,000, it also seemed that keeping the daily tally below 1,000 at the peak was a political necessity. On 10 April the *Guardian* reported that the peak number of deaths had been reached at 980, with the death of another NHS doctor, Dr Fayez's Ayache, a Suffolk GP. Ten weeks later the same paper drew attention to the fact that in reality the death toll had passed 1000 on 22 consecutive days with the actual peak having come on 8 April when 1,445 people perished.

An additional major scandal came with the realisation that no attempt had been made to count or recognise the hundreds of COVID deaths occurring among frontline clinical staff, many of whom turned out to have Black, Asian and Minority Ethnic backgrounds. This was compounded disastrously when a report into the possible reasons for these latter deaths by Professor Kevin Fenton was submitted to the government but emerged with the recommendations for action redacted.

The numbers game

The misleading nature of the press conference statistics was not confined to their incomplete nature. Timeliness was also an issue. Quite remarkably, in a country that can claim to have been publishing weekly Bills of Mortality based on the parish registration of deaths as described in Daniel Defoe's account of the London Plague in 1722, and later carried in *The Times* newspaper, the same thing was not possible in the age of the computer. In particular it seemed that counting those who had died was not something that either the hospitals or Public Health England could do at the weekend. The obfuscation caused by the daily numbers confused those accustomed to working with data as much as the lay public.

In late June, with the end of the lockdown looming and with the first example of a second wave in Leicester, the extent of the continuing dysfunction of the numbers game became apparent. According to the government data available to the city council the total of cases for the whole month had been 145. On 30 June on the basis of 800 cases known centrally but not to the field a further lockdown was required by PHE to the frustration and annoyance of the local leaders who had been kept in the dark as a result of yet more data hoarding by PHE.

With so-called 'Independence Day', 4 July, when the lockdown would end, and large parts of the population in party mode, stimulated by Johnson's new slogan of 'Spend, Spend, spend', around the country local authorities and Directors of Public Health were waking up to the realisation that they had been systematically misled by a government hell-bent on getting the numbers under the wire in time to reboot the economy on the appointed day.

As well as miscounting and sleight of hand, over-counting, over-claiming and underdelivering were all par for the course. Despite large numbers of PPE deliveries being claimed frontline staff still reported extensive shortages. Extravagant claims were made for the testing capacity for the virus with health secretary Matt Hancock setting a target of 100,000 tests per day by the end of April. This target was apparently magically reached in the last few days of the month, but turned out to be a concoction that included tests that were mailed out for people to use at home and never returned, tests that were returned but could not be processed, were missing labels or badly taken and tests that were sent out in large batches to care homes with many times more kits than the homes had patients. Tests carried out by the NHS turned out to be much more reliable than those carried out by the private sector contractor Deloitte.

Local intelligence, public-health centralisation, and the loss of the public-health observatories
Sound and timely intelligence is the basis of effective public health action. The tension between blue skies and esoteric academic research and practical action is one that many public-health systems struggle with. It is one that is not helped by the bias of the British university funding system that rewards pure research to the detriment of what used to be called 'extension' or research that focused on putting evidence into practice.

In the early nineteen eighties this issue came to a head in Liverpool where the health authorities, fed up with bankrolling the medical school for research in which the academics took the money and disappeared for three or four years, coming back with the answer to the research question when the question had changed, collectively funded the first Public Health Observatory. The terms of reference were to produce timely, action-orientated intelligence which could respond to local and regional public-health questions in the north west with 'good enough' science and a timescale of weeks or months rather than years.

Over the following 20 years the Observatory established itself as a vital source of intelligence within the region, able to hold and handle data sets from a variety of agencies, including those containing sensitive personal information, in real time, and complement it with *ad hoc* surveys and research.

Following the 1999 Public Health white paper, Minister of Public Health, Tessa Jowell and Chief Medical Officer Sir Liam Donaldson were so impressed with the experience of the Liverpool Observatory that regional observatories were established around the country and others were established inter-nationally. In the following years these observatories made significant contributions to public health in England at local, regional and national levels and beyond. Tragically following the establishment of PHE they were closed down and replaced by a centralised Knowledge Information Team under the direction of John Newton. There is little doubt that if the regional Observatories had been kept the intelligence disasters and opaque data of COVID-19 in the UK would have been much less likely. In particular there would have been no grounds for Public Health England's defence against their data hoarding of personal clinical information rather than sharing detailed local data with Directors of Public Health.

The politics get dirty
Famously, during the Thatcher government in the 1980's when the Prime Minister asked Lord Sainsbury to review the NHS, he is reported to have said that if Florence Nightingale was to review it she would ask who was in charge. His report led to the intro-

duction of general management. Similarly while those responsible for leading the UK response to COVID made error after error, for much of the time it was unclear as to who was meant to be in charge. Even when the Prime Minister was present this was the case and he was reported to have asked the question himself of his civil servants.

Dysfunction between Ministers, department of health officials, the NHS, and PHE lay behind and contributed to many of the problems. Whether it was a question of a clear vision and strategy for action, procurement of tests, reagents, PPE, and oxygen; the decision to discharge large numbers of untested patients to care homes, the decision to create the 4,000 bed Nightingale hospital out of the Exel conference centre and then be unable to staff it, the data hoarding and data mismanagement. The whole system failed.

So too did the main public-health organisations and bodies that sat on their hands until late in the emergency, together with some of the individual public-health leaders, too close to Public Health England and the patrons of power, influence, patronage and honours to exercise the advocacy for the public health that is in their stewardship. The most generous assessment is that they had flawed judgement.

For those who put their heads above the parapets, the politics became dirty. Following the Panorama programme exposing the failure to act on the Cygnus exercise in 2016, the unsafe practices of recycling out of date PPE, and the cynical double counting of gloves and other garments and downgrading of the threat posed by the COVID virus, a campaign began to discredit voices critical of the government as if criticism was morally wrong. Those who took part in the programme were labelled as political extremists and efforts made to blacklist them from the BBC. Emilie Maitlis and other broadcasters and commentators were targeted, especially by extremist agitators like Guido Fawkes. I found myself the focus of accusations of anti-Semitism in an attempt to have me blacklisted by the BBC. They were entirely spurious, but it showed how low the cabinet would stoop to sabotage a fair discussion of its governance of Britain.

15

Lockdown

When the lockdown came in the UK on 26 March it was arguably two to three weeks too late in the communities that were affected, such as London with half the number of known infections in Britain on 16 March. Those people who would become sick and die as the epidemic reached its peak, during the first weeks of April, would have been infected earlier in March. During that period the government had been vacillating, whilst maintaining that it was 'following the science'. Its politically-led messaging continued to produce a cluster of superlatives about how 'world beating' the country was, simultaneously casting doubt on the value of the measures that other countries had been taking. Sadly its advisers did nothing to disabuse the public of these misleading claims, whilst behind the scenes those others who were supposedly feeding 'the science' remained anonymous within the vague and arcane advisory umbrella of SAGE. After the sudden change of direction on 16 March, when Neil Ferguson's modellers appeared to recognise that they had been on the wrong track and the Chief Medical Officer's four point plan crumbled to be replaced by 'suppression', it took 10 crucial and ambiguous days before explicit action was put in place.

The lack of systematic and large scale community testing for the virus had meant that policy-making and action was being planned in the dark in the absence of detailed local knowledge of the incidence, prevalence and spread of the virus. None of this had made any difference to the bluff and bluster of the announcements coming from the government in its press conferences and passively endorsed by its key advisors and other members of the SAGE committees. When lockdown finally came, together with the suspension of most of the activities of everyday life, it was trailing public opinion and seemingly over-influenced by specialist behavioural-science advisors who postulated that if it was done too soon the public would tire of it and it would be unable to make it stick.

The narrow behavioural disciplinary base of this advice in psychology, rather than including anthropology, overlooked how people actually live their lives, rather than relying on laboratory theories and experiments. This had relevance to particular groups, including faith communities, VIPs and younger people and exposed the failure to fully engage with the public in open and transparent ways. There was an increasing public awareness of being treated paternalistically as children by the cabinet. The public was also being treated as a homogeneous group with no recognition of the importance of demographics, values and cultural aspects that might influence the behaviours of particular groups.

This lack of an understanding of the 'lived experience' of people had been behind the lost weeks in the Ebola epidemic in West Africa when a narrow medical mindset failed to grasp the importance of the role of village women's committees in the intimate body washing rituals of the dead. It was only when it was realised that the village women's committees, rather than the male chiefs, were the key to changing the deeply entrenched and intimate ritual practices which was necessary to improve biosecurity and prevent the transmission of infection that effective interventions became possible. Sadly this learning, together with the growing recognition of the central importance of community trust, that was so in evidence after the Grenfell Tower tragedy, was another casualty of the neglect of pandemic and emergency planning since 2013. It would later be profoundly affected by the perceived hypocrisy of VIPs breaking the lockdown.

Implementing lockdown and social distancing
As a species we are risk taking animals, but we resent either risks or constraints being imposed on us by others. In the film Superman the Movie, after rescuing her from a helicopter crash, Superman tells Lois Lane that flying is still the safest way to travel. That many people are more frightened of flying than driving their own car, which is much more dangerous, is down to the sense of control that comes from being behind the wheel yourself. Concepts such as locus of control and sense of coherence are at the heart of the practice of health promotion as a key vehicle for protecting and improving public health. When it comes to legislative or other government interventions to protect its citizens we are party to an unwritten contract in which we trade off some part of our freedom for the benefit of increased personal and family safety.

In invoking the Public Health (Control of Disease) Act 1984, without primary legislation, following the quarantining of Wuhan returnees in February, the Johnson government was tacitly accepting this responsibility, but had failed to follow through with openness and public engagement. These qualities were essential for the maintenance of trust and adherence to the requirements of the lockdown, including 2 metres social spacing between individual non-family household members. These measures were a prerequisite for suppressing an epidemic that was out of control by reducing the 'Re' number and protecting those most vulnerable to infection, serious complications, and death. The loss of trust that was oozing away, along with the government handling off the emergency, would make it that much more difficult to sustain the integrity of the lockdown.

Shielding and reducing the spread those at most risk
On 29 March, amid conflicting claims from government advisers about the potential death toll, the *Observer* reported that the prime minister would be writing to 30 million households warning everybody that the coronavirus outbreak was likely to worsen and he would be prepared to tighten the lockdown which had just come into play. The letter would make explicit the government's orders on symptoms, social distancing and hand washing as ministers battled to prepare the NHS for the coming onslaught. 'from the start we have sought to put in the right measures at the right time' according to Johnson.

According to an Opinium poll at this point the vast majority of voters (92%), backed the lockdown with 57% thinking that the lockdown measures did not go far enough and 56% thinking that the government had not acted fast enough. Nevertheless approval for the government's handling of the crisis was also growing.

The intention behind the encouragement of social distancing and the more formal instigation of household lockdown was to reduce the levels of the circulating virus and to protect the most vulnerable. These groups were initially identified from the experience in China as older people (over 60 or 70 years of age, with the highest risk being among the most elderly groups) together with those suffering from particular long-term conditions.

Rigid shielding was proposed for those at greatest risk, totalling over two million people, who would be required to stay strictly at home for the duration prescribed by the government. After some delay a letter went to all general practitioners on 9 April requesting that they identify all their patients at highest clinical risk from COVID-19, who would be asked to stay at home and avoid face to face contact for twelve weeks. This was to cover a range of patients including those with specific cancers, a variety of chronic respiratory conditions, metabolic disorders, those who were immunosuppressed, suffering from particular congenital abnormalities and pregnant women. It later became apparent that obesity, rather than being important because of its association with type II or maturity-onset diabetes, was actually a risk factor in its own right. A high proportion of those who died from the virus were overweight or obese, irrespective of their diabetic status, a phenomenon that seemed to be associated with the pathological and replication processes initiated by the virus in fat tissue.

Although the behavioural scientist advisers to SAGE had warned about potential difficulties in securing long-term public compliance, the initial response was high, as reflected in dramatic reductions in road traffic levels, empty streets and reduced footfall at the shops that remained open. Some early indications of the fault lines that would later develop came in reports of day trippers flocking to rural beauty spots including open spaces, beaches, and the National Parks. In some areas, such as the Lake District and the Yorkshire Dales, they where met with a hostile response from local residents and there were reports of the police using their new powers to turn them away. Derbyshire police were accused of overreacting by using drones to monitor outsiders and issuing on-the-spot fines, whilst Deputy Chief Medical Officer Jennie Harries confirmed that police were correct to stop people driving to places to exercise. These interventions led former Supreme Court Judge Lord Sumption to claim that the UK was in danger of becoming a 'police state'.

By 31 March, less than a week after lockdown, the Chief Scientific Adviser claimed that social distancing was working, with the NHS coping as numbers stopped accelerating. This was an odd claim in view of how recently the lockdown had been put in place compared with the incubation period of the virus, the poor data available about the prevalence of the virus in the community and the fact that deaths were still to peak over a week later. It would also later emerge that not all COVID patients were now being admitted to hospital following the adoption by general practitioners and hospital consultants of the Rockford Index, a screening tool that claimed to identify those patients too frail to benefit from hospital care.

Earlier in the emergency concern had begun to be expressed that the pandemic might be causing increases in stress and anxiety, particularly among those with existing mental health problems such as obsessive compulsive disorders. Difficulties in sleeping, feelings of sadness, anger and helplessness, phobias of contact with others, physical symptoms and self-harm were among the issues being widely reported and discussed. Agencies were recording large increases in reports of domestic violence. Two weeks into the lockdown there was growing concern about the mental health of those experiencing social isolation, potentially in vulnerable environments, and *The Times* reported that nine people had died in a string of suspected domestic killings, including a family of three living in Hemel Hempstead, and a family of four in Sussex.

Love in the time of COVID
For many older people with longstanding health problems, who were in supportive relationships, some sense of security was to be found in being shielded at home. Lockdown was much more problematic for many younger people at the time of life when they are exploring the world and embarking on the excitement of new relationships. For them this all ground to a halt in March as schools and universities were disrupted and many young workers were furloughed. Dr Jennie Harries warning to couples living in separate residences of the dangers of spreading infections by visiting each other did not deter Professor Neil Ferguson, whose

married lover, Antonia Staats travelled across London to visit him at his home, leading to his resignation from the SAGE committee. Dr Harries suggested that couples should consider moving in with each other for the duration of the lockdown, something that may have been a less disruptive option for Antonia Staats and Professor Ferguson, who was reported to be living apart from his wife.

Mainstream media reported that there was a big increase in online and virtual dating sites with advice being given by some pundits that 'the safest sexual partner in the lockout is yourself'. Undoubtedly this was a frustrating time for young people whose hormones were in full flow and many of them were to need little prompting to break the lockdown once mixed messages began to be issued by celebrities and those in leadership positions. Many of the difficulties faced by this group might have been avoided had large scale, frequent testing been available, offering them the opportunity to be billeted with other young people, essential and frontline workers and volunteers in communal settings, such as requisitioned hotels, boarding houses and university halls of residence, separate from those needing to shield, provided that they were regularly tested. As late as the summer months this level of testing was still not available and despite a call from NHS Chief Executive, Simon Stevens, for NHS staff to be tested twice weekly, as was the case with premiership footballers, who had resumed the 2019-20 season games, the government rejected the idea and voted against it in the House of Commons.

Faith communities
One characteristic of many religious faiths is their commitment to collective worship and to pilgrimage. As early as February this had been identified as potentially problematic in Bahrain, with regard to the religious pilgrimages made to the holy sites in Iran by Shi'ite Muslims and these were cancelled together with Friday prayers in

all mosques. Despite the good control achieved over the pandemic in Bahrain, the religious month of Ramadan, which is characterised by fasting, prayer, reflection and community celebrations raised issues of a breakdown of social distancing with a subsequent spike in cases. Increases in cases among Muslim communities were also reported in the UK and from other places, including Melbourne, Australia, where concerns were raised about the stigmatisation of Muslims, and India where the arrival of the pandemic was blamed on Muslims, by the majority Hindu population.

This phenomenon was also to be found among other faith groups with a cluster reported in *The Times* on 21 March from a church in Wolverhampton. In March, reports from South Korea that the initial fast growing epidemic was linked to the congregational practices of a religious sect in the city of Daegu led to recriminations and the threat of legal action against its leader. In the Church of England the closure of the churches by church leaders proved controversial.

In the *Guardian* of 30 June it was reported that Jewish burials between March and May were 127% higher than the same time in 2019. It was suggested that the Jewish community had suffered 2.5 times as many deaths as a result of the pandemic than the non-Jewish community. The Office of National Statistics published data showing that the mortality rate was higher for Muslims, Jews, Hindus and Sikhs than for Christians or those of no religion. Celebrations to mark the Jewish festival of Purim, in early March, which is characterised by large celebratory congregations involved in singing and dancing, were thought to have contributed to the spread of the virus in the Jewish population.

VIPs

Viruses are blind to administrative boundaries and to social class, although after the initial UK cases appear to have been among the

187

skiing classes, the pandemic went on to make a greater impact in the poorer areas of the country and among Black, Asian and Minority Ethnic groups. That VIP's might be deserving of separate consideration, resulting from their special place in the universe and the belief that the rules for others did not apply to them, could be concluded from the behaviours of a succession of celebrities, as a result of which some of them became infected with the virus.

The prime minister's sister Rachel later admitted to commuting between her London home and her property in the West Country, Labour MP, Stephen Kinnock, visited his father, the former Labour Party leader Neil to celebrate his birthday, Scotland Chief Medical Officer, Catherine Calderwood was forced to resign after making two visits with her family to their holiday cottage from Edinburgh, the Housing, Communities and Local Government Minister, Robert Jenrick, was forced to explain himself when he travelled 150 miles from his London to his Shropshire home, several professional footballers were caught having parties with sex workers in hotels, royals Zara and Mike Tyndall insisted that they would not self isolate after skiing in a coronavirus hotspot in Northern Italy. Notoriously Dominic Cummings took himself and his family off to his parent's house in Durham, whilst suffering from the virus and visited Barnard Castle, 16 miles away, on his wife's birthday to check whether his vision was good enough to drive back to London. Numerous other examples of non-compliance were reported from other leading figures from communities around the country, arousing anger from the general public.

Masks

> You that hide behind walls
> You that hide behind desks

I just want you to know
I can see through your masks
Bob Dylan, 1963

From the beginning of the pandemic in the UK the government had been keen to stress their adherence to 'the science' that was being provided by a largely secret set of experts advising it via the SAGE committees. That this science was not only narrowly drawn, but also often flawed and not much more than opinion being dressed up as facts, would contribute to the erosion of trust and eventually the establishment of an 'Independent SAGE' under the chairmanship of the highly respected former Chief Scientific Adviser, Sir David King. Some of the 'Facts' that didn't stack up included:

* *Testing and Contact tracing.* In a country with such a robust and resilient public-health system, it was said that the WHO Director General's instruction to 'test, test, test', was an irrelevance, applicable only to underdeveloped countries. The truth was very different. We no longer had the capacity to test and trace because of Andrew Lansley's disastrous reforms of 2013 and the centralisation of PHE together with the outsourcing of services to the private sector that had stripped bare the capacity of local and regional public-health teams to fulfil their mission.
* *Personal Protective Equipment.* Unique to the UK it had been decided to downgrade the risk of the virus from a 'High Consequence Infectious Disease' requiring full personal protection for those in clinically exposed roles to 'HG3'. This enabled the government to pass off the failure to maintain supplies of protective equipment for major incidents as irrelevant in the face of a less serious viral threat.
Discharge of thousands of infected hospital patients to care

189

homes, starting a second, parallel epidemic, that would kill thousands. This was presented as a misunderstanding and a misrepresentation—that no clinician would have knowingly done that—despite evidence that on March 17, NHS England had sent a letter advising hospitals to discharge patients to 'free up the maximum inpatient and critical care capacity', whilst at the same time there was no guidance requiring patients to be tested for COVID-19 before they were sent to care homes. Later, on 4 July, Professor Paul Johnstone, national director at PHE, would be quoted as saying that 'Care homes have always been a priority for government and PHE continues to work closely with care homes and the social care sector to provide advice and support to them in preventing and managing cases and outbreaks. All of PHE's advice and guidance is based on the latest scientific evidence.' May be, but it didn't add up.

* *Allowing Mass Gatherings* to take place in Bristol, Cheltenham, at Anfield, and elsewhere, in the week of 9 March, on the grounds that people at such gatherings are in contact for a short time, insufficient to spread the virus. By 4 July, with new cases of infection still running in the hundreds daily and with a new lockdown in Leicester, the Chief Scientific Adviser Sir Patrick Vallance, who had been opposed to preventing social gatherings in march, was telling *The Times* that pubs could become 'super spreading environments' if social distancing rules were ignored.

* The *Delay in Local Lockdowns* in March on the grounds that the public would tire of it and it would be difficult to make it stick. Despite treating the public as children from the beginning of the emergency the level of compliance had been extremely high but sadly too late to prevent thousands of deaths. According to Sir David King, many of these could have been saved if lockdowns had been introduced earlier.

These inconsistencies, of opinion dressed up as science, and of politically led science rather than scientifically informed policy loomed especially large with the controversial role of the wearing of masks and face coverings in public places to reduce viral transmission. A recurring theme in the handling of the pandemic had been the apparent unwillingness of both the government and its advisers to recommend interventions that had been tried and found useful elsewhere in preventing, containing, mitigating and otherwise responding to the enormity of this threat to life and health. Nowhere had this been more in evidence than in the approach to mask wearing, a practice that has long been widespread in many parts of the world in the face of respiratory infections.

The corona group of viruses, of which COVID-19 is a member, are spread in exhaled breath and coughs of children and adults in the aerosol form of droplets. They may also be spread by the faecal-oral route as a result of gastrointestinal infection, a factor likely to be especially important in children, and in the frail elderly especially if suffering from incontinence or dementia, where poor hygiene may be especially prominent. In addition COVID-19 virus may live on hard surfaces for up to 72 hours.

On 12 March, as the public debate about the value of wearing masks was gathering momentum and sales were rocketing, Dr Harries warned that members of the public could be placing themselves at risk by wearing face masks; she went on to claim that the masks could 'actually trap the virus' and cause the person wearing it to become infected.

At the beginning of the COVID pandemic, while it was possible to claim that detailed evidence of the effectiveness of face masks and coverings was uncertain, both citizen science of lived experience together with actual published research, including that from the Spanish 'flu, lent support to mask wearing. During the 1918-19 pandemic, Boston researchers had demonstrated lower case fatality rates in open-air hospitals with natural ventilation and gauze masks and Dr Hood, the physician superintendent at the Marylebone hospital in London had demonstrated a similar effect with lint masks. A systematic review of the English language literature on the prevention of transmission of the Influenza virus in 2009 found that while there was some evidence to support the wearing of masks during illness to reduce virus transmission, there was little evidence to support the use of masks or respirators to prevent becoming infected and the review argued that further studies were needed. That review was over 10 years ago and research published in *Nature Science* in March 2020 concluded that surgical masks may help prevent infected people from making others sick with seasonal viruses. WHO would in August change its guidance on masks from neutral to recommending that wearing masks be extended to children over 12 in high-risk areas and that those over 60 wear a medical grade mask to prevent airborne and droplet infection from COVID.

The reasons for initial British opposition to masks and face coverings seemed difficult to understand, given the growing evidence base and experience from other countries and their accelerating adoption elsewhere. Part of the explanation may lie in a flawed approach to science by advisers who seemed to imply that no evidence of effect is evidence of none, or of negative effect. It may also be bound up in the 'Little Englander' mentality of 'exceptionalism' and the repeated rhetoric about the UK having the best science in the world when a little modesty might have served us better.

Other cultural factors may also have been in play too it having been suggested that British male identity may be too fragile to cope with mask wearing. In contrast in Asia, where sneezing in public is unacceptable, it is a deeply engrained part of culture and social etiquette that may have its origins in the pandemic of 1918/9 and may also reflect some residual adherence to nineteenth century miasma theory that stressed the air-borne nature of disease in contrast to the more western fear of contagion through touch.

However, as with the March change of pathogen status from High Impact Infectious Disease to HG3, made necessary by the shortage of PPE, the most likely explanation of the government's initial intransigence on the subject of masks was probably the fear that the market would be unable to meet public demand if their wearing became commonplace. In June, as the economic imperative of easing up on the lockdown came to dominate the agenda and it became ever clearer that science was secondary, the U-turn to embrace facial coverings in public was adopted without a second take. By then the market had geared up and large quantities of masks and face coverings were freely available. This was too late for the many bus and taxi drivers who had become victims of the virus together with others in people facing public service roles.

16

The Forgotten

What distinguishes the practise of public health from that of the clinical professions is the focus on whole populations and groups as distinct from one on individuals and families. In this it is the denominator that is all important and it is the starting point for any comparisons of experience or outcome. In constructing these denominators the work of the Victorian public-health pioneers can be summarised as *registration* (of births and deaths), *notification* (of infectious disease), and *advice* (to central government, local authorities, and to the public).

One of the challenges to practitioners is to make visible those populations and groups for whom no ready-made denominators can be drawn down or readily found, those people whom the World Health Organization tends to classify as 'underserved groups', and who may not be registered with statutory agencies. These groups may include, the homeless, rough sleepers, itinerants and illegal migrants, commercial sex workers, drug users, and others who live on the fringes of mainstream society. Others include those who by virtue of their lifestyles, medical or living conditions may themselves be at risk or may pose a risk to others but not be on the radar of those best placed to respond to their needs. In addition children and adults who may be especially vulnerable, include the disabled, those subject to domestic abuse or children in care, those older people in care homes, those in prison or other forms of judicial custody.

The failure to implement routine testing of those in hospital environments, together with the major problems of provision of PPE meant that hospitals themselves were becoming contaminated environments, putting all those in them at potential risk.

80-year-old Marita Edwards, a retired cleaner was the first victim, dying in Newport's Royal Gwent Hospital after a routine gall bladder operation on 28 February. In addition to the various at-risk groups it became clear that NHS frontline workers themselves and especially those from Black, Asian and Minority Ethnic groups were at especial risk and a matter of concern that those monitoring the pandemic were initially unable to give up to the minute details of their tragic deaths or be transparent about the probable reasons for them being put in harm's way. The first NHS doctors to be reported as victims of COVID-19, Mr Amgen El-Hawrani, an ENT surgeon from Leicester, and Mr Adil El Tayar, an organ transplant specialist from the West Middlesex University Hospital, were both of a BAME background.

When dealing with a highly contagious and potentially fatal novel virus such as COVID-19 it is the responsibility of public-health agencies to be sighted on all of these and even if they don't have direct control over protective interventions, to be in a position to provide advice and assurance that such interventions are being attended to. Of these the position of those in care homes proved to be especially problematic whilst that of prisoners and prison officers appeared to be shrouded in secrecy while that of other groups ranged from having some intelligence to next to none.

Residents of care homes and their carers
The concern about care homes was to mushroom as the epidemic curve in the UK escalated, especially after it became clear that the

government had only been announcing confirmed hospital deaths in the press conferences. According to Andrew Grice, writing in the *Independent*, whilst health secretary Matt Hancock claimed on 28 April that government support for care homes had been 'absolutely at the front of mind right from the start' and the Chief Scientific Adviser, Sir Patrick Vallance had said that SAGE, which first discussed the outbreak in January, had warned 'very early on' about the risk to care homes, the reality was again very different. Because of the primary focus on hospitals and the political fear of them falling over, care homes had taken a back seat until the steadily climbing toll of deaths among both residents and care home workers forced it onto governments attention. By this time it was too late to prevent many more deaths.

The governments initial guidance, which lasted until Friday 13 March claimed that it was 'very unlikely people receiving care in a care home or the community will become infected'. It was to be a month later, in mid-April, that Hancock would announce a new package of measures to support care home staff and residents as well as procedures to allow people to say goodby to loved ones. At the same time the Secretary of State revealed a new 'care' badge, described as a 'badge of honour', for social care workers so they could get the same public recognition as NHS staff, for whom the general public had begun a Thursday night ritual of coming out onto the street to clap. Hancock was widely ridiculed for his gesture of the badge, which was both trivial and an insulting irrelevance.

The situation in the care homes was intimately bound up with both the continuing failure of PHE to ramp up COVID-19 antigen testing to detect the levels and distribution of the virus both in the community and in at risk frontline workers and settings, and the immense pressure that was building on the NHS with the numbers of sick patients beginning to be referred. By mid-March the advisers to Sage had been predicting that over 4%

of the public were likely to be infected with the virus, leading to two million hospital admissions, whilst the NHS had only 100,000 acute beds. It was predicted that the Intensive Care Units in London would be imminently overwhelmed, with an indication from several hospitals that they were on the edge. It was at this point that large numbers of non-corona, elderly hospital patients, who were deemed fit for transfer, were moved out into care homes without being tested for the virus. In the event, the Nightingale hospitals were not needed. In addition some beds in childrens beds around the country were freed up for COVID-19 patients.

Although it was widely reported that these discharges were responsible for the parallel COVID epidemic in care homes, this is disputed by Simon Stevens, the Chief Executive of NHS England, who maintains that in reality the number of discharges to care homes in this period in 2020 was less than in previous years.

In any event the other possible explanation for care home infection lies in the fragmented and unsatisfactory nature of the care home sector, split between large chains funded with offshore private equity and dependent on a business model involving low pay, poor terms and conditions, low morale and the risky movement of staff between homes, and the smaller family run businesses, often with highly motivated and loyal staff who moved into the care homes themselves for the lockdown to care for their patients. It is estimated that two thirds of the large chain homes became infected compared with only two in five of the family businesses. Some individual care homes had large numbers of deaths with 15 being reported from Oak Springs in Wavertree, Liverpool, (15 April), 10 at Home Farm Care Home on the Isle of Skye.(20 May), and 24 at Melbury Court (2 June).

By 3 July the *New Scientist* magazine was reporting that 19,394 people were confirmed to have died from COVID-19 in care homes across England and Wales according to new data from the Office of National Statistics, which had also estimated that one in every five people living in care homes had become infected with cases in at least 56% of all care homes. 7% of all care home staff were estimated to have had coronavirus since the beginning of the pandemic.

After five months of the emergency it was now finally possible to produce these figures as a result of sample surveys being carried out into more than 5,000 care homes. Care-home residents over 65 years of age and those with dementia would receive a test every 28 days and staff every week. That this had not happened earlier was as a result of decisions taken by PHE together with health secretary Hancock and Chief Medical Officer Whitty, on the basis of the lack of testing capacity and the need to choose priorities. The choice to focus testing on intensive care and emergency admissions to confirm diagnoses, rather than using clinical criteria and freeing up testing capacity for testing those at risk, entrants into the country and routine sampling to enable local public-health teams to better focus their tracing and isolating efforts is one worthy of further scrutiny.

Looking back over the pandemic on 4 July, Professor Brian Jarman told *The Times* that health chiefs had been aware of rising numbers of coronavirus cases in care homes even as hospitals had been told to discharge patients without tests. Data on 'acute respiratory outbreaks' in care homes from PHE showed that cases began to climb rapidly in the week to March 20, with 249 outbreaks that week compared with 41 a week earlier. When NHS England had written to hospitals advising them to discharge patients, there was no guidance advising them to test patients before they were sent to care homes. According to Jarman 'they watched unfolding events like Roman spectators watching gladiators 'thrown to the lions'. In response, Professor Paul Johnson stated that 'All of PHE's advice and guidance is based on the latest scientific evidence'.

Prisons

COVID-19 is what public-health professionals used to call a 'crowd disease'. It thrives wherever people congregate in conditions in which exhaled clouds of virus particles, whether as droplet transmission through close contact, or in smaller particles as aerosols over longer distances, can find entry to another person. When the first two cases were identified at the hotel in York, in January, PHE said that being less than two metres apart for 15 minutes was sufficient to place people at risk of catching the coronavirus.

Closed communities of one kind and another are particularly risky environments and the consequences of failing to maintain biosecurity of both the environment and through personal protection, backed up by extensive testing, tracking and isolating, had led to thousands of unnecessary deaths in hospitals and care homes. Prisons and other custodial institutions represent an additional sector carrying especially high risk of virus transmission, not least because many of the older, Victorian prisons are overcrowded and even in normal times have environments where hygienic standards are difficult to maintain. Early outbreaks of COVID in prisons in China and Iran, where 85,000 prisoners had been released, had alerted the world to the dangers they posed and both these countries had embarked on large scale early release of prisoners as a precautionary measure, as had Bahrain and some others. When the virus took root in the UK, it looked as if this enlightened measure might be one that would be implemented here too.

In March—following the first death in prison related to COVID-19 of 48-year-old Brian Moore at HMP Peterborough—Lord Chancellor Robert Buckland, announced that 4,000 low risk offenders in England and Wales, whose sentences were nearing an end, could expect to be released on licence. This proposal proved to be short lived. In a Victorian turn that undermined protection for prison staff, prime minister Johnson refused to sanction the release of thousands of low-risk prisoners, according to *The Times* of 31 March, whilst agreeing to the release of about 50 expectant mothers as they were classified as vulnerable.

Meanwhile, all family visits to prisons had been suspended on 24 March. By 31 May The *Guardian* would report that 'some children are allowed out of their cells for just 40 minutes each day with family visits and education drastically curtailed' and the Children's Commissioner for England was warning of the increased risk of injury and self-harm among young offenders and those in other custodial institutions. During this time other measures to reduce mixing among the 80,000 incarcerated prisoners were introduced. These included minimising social interaction in workshops, classrooms, canteens, gymnasia, and communal showers with prisoners being confined to their cells for over 23 hours each day. At HMP Wandsworth, where 52 prisoners had been classified as infected, prisoners who had COVID symptoms were placed in the same cells as those who had tested positive for the virus, an approach known as 'co-hosting'. According to the *Guardian* on 31 March there were no plans for further testing at the gaol and prisoners who displayed symptoms would be placed on the isolation wing. The Prison Reform Trust commented that PHE had reported that 'access to testing for prisoners has been variable and limited 'and suggested that the number of confirmed cases could not be taken as a true reflection of the extent of those infected.

A press release from the Ministry of Justice on 28 April said that 'jails are successfully limiting deaths and the transmission of the virus within the estate'. By the end of April the *Guardian* was reporting that, with a likelihood of more than 2,000 cases, the deaths of 15 prisoners and 5 prison officers could be directly or indirectly linked to the virus with some sources suggesting more. As of 12 May, 404 cases were being reported among prisoners by the House of Commons Library together with the deaths of 21 prisoners and 7 members of the prisons staff.

As the virus continued its progress through the prisons, the limited early release programme had barely started and in a statement on 27 April the Justice Secretary admitted that progress had been slow. On 12 May the prisons minister, Lucy Fraser, reported that a total of 81 prisoners had been released in England and Wales during lockdown- 55 on temporary release, 21 because they were pregnant, and 5 on compassionate grounds. PHE was mostly silent on the issues affecting the prisoners, their inmates and the prison officers despite the duty of care which they hold over these vulnerable populations. Remarkably it adopted a self-congratulatory tone in a department-of-justice analysis that reported worryingly high levels of COVID-19 infection despite admitting that prison staff had much more access to testing than did the prisoners.

In the absence of a robust and inclusive approach to testing among residents and workers in the prisons it is very difficult to make an informed judgement as to how well this population's human rights, health and wellbeing, were protected. In the absence of clear transparency—another instance of the Johnson cabinet's secretive approach to data—it is not possible to be confident about the total numbers of COVID-19 deaths being acknowledged, whether potential victims are being considered by coroners and whether, in the absence of complete prisoner testing, some measure of excess deaths may be a more reliable indicator.

On 30 June, in response to Parliamentary Questions from Lord David Alton, the government response was that 'As of Friday 12 June, we are aware of 495 prisoner and 963 prison staff COVID-19 cases across England and Wales. These figures reflect the cumulative numbers of recorded positive cases—not the number of live cases—of COVID-19 and include individuals that have since recovered. As of 12 June, 23 prisoners and 9 members of prison staff have sadly died having tested positive or shown symptoms. The restricted regimes introduced to protect prisoners and staff from COVID-19 mean that prisoners are spending longer in their cells than normal which raises new and different risks to safety and mental health of prisoners'.

Some of these numbers appear to be incomplete and require further attention. The number of prisoners in England and Wales in 2020 was just under 81,000 and the number of prison officers in 2019 was just over 23,000. Given that the testing of prison officers was much more complete than that for prisoners, then a minimum estimate for the numbers of cases among the prisoners might be around 4 x that for the prison officers, or 4 x 963, perhaps 4,000. Assuming that ascertainment of cause of death would have been more accurate among prison officers, (9/963, or approximately 1%) as they were being systematically tested, the same proportionate mortality among prisoners would lead us to expect that around 40 prisoner deaths could be attributed to the COVID virus. In reality other factors will have been in play including the generally poorer health status of prisoners and less access to specialist medical care compared to prison officers, factors that would lead to an anticipated higher mortality rate among prisoners. Collateral damage from this secondary epidemic in the nations prisons may also have been leakage of the virus from prison officers, infecting family members together with further epidemic seeding in the absence of systematic community testing and tracing.

17

Dying Matters

It is estimated that between 50-100 million people died worldwide during the 1918-19 pandemic of influenza. 800 people perished in China during the 2002 outbreak of SARS (the nearest virus relative to COVID-19 yet identified); 17,000 in the Swine 'flu pandemic worldwide of 2009; 11,000 in the Ebola outbreak in West Africa in 2014. About 32 million people are estimated to have died from HIV worldwide since the beginning of the pandemic in the early 1980's, and between 290,000 and 650,000 die each year from seasonal influenza.

Each year, globally, over 3 million people die from alcohol and 750,000 from drug related conditions; 1.5 million people from tuberculosis, 1.3 million in road traffic accidents, and 400,00 each from malaria and homicide. Some estimates suggest that up to 10% of all deaths are the result of the adverse effects of medical treatment.

Every year worldwide there are about 58 million deaths, of which around 50% are of people aged over 70. Some commentators have suggested that during the current pandemic of COVID-19 the international response has been an over-reaction when compared with the statistics from other forms of viral and infectious disease or external causes and that as many of those who have perished 'didn't have long to go anyway' we were making too much of it.

As quoted in *Metro*, journalist Jeremy Warner writing in the *Daily Telegraph* on March 3 had claimed that 'not to put too fine a point on it, from an entirely disinterested economic perspective, the COVID-19 might even prove mildly beneficial in the long term by disproportionately culling elderly dependents'. Warner's callous sentiments provoked a strong backlash with readers describing them as 'despicable' and 'deeply sinister'. He later said that on reflection he should not have used the word 'cull'.

Understanding and making sense of these statistics of the risks of everyday life and death is not simple. Getting to grips with the risks themselves involves risk assessment, risk communication and risk management together with the measurement of outcome. Each of these has been badly handled in the UK, either through incompetence, inadequate systems, or attempts at political manipulation. Whilst each of these aspects is important in evaluating the response to COVID-19, at the heart of the matter are our personal values.

Perhaps what is most important is that everything is relative unless until it involves a relative. As the late medical statistician, Professor Major Greenwood, of the London School of Hygiene and Tropical Medicine put it many years ago 'Statistics are patients with the tears wiped off'. It is notable that after the HIV virus first began to affect the stigmatised population of gay men in developed countries there was little interest in responding to it or researching it until it began to affect women and children, straight men and people who were deemed by some to be 'innocent'. Similarly there was little interest in the Ebola virus, which had been identified at the same time as HIV in West Africa, so long as it affected only poor and marginalised populations; that all changed once it had spilled over into westerners.

Planning for pandemic death

The earlier planning documents for pandemic influenza from the Cabinet Office with their guidance for local planners provided the basic assumptions that came into play with the first indication of the COVID pandemic. These assumptions, which were modified as the real nature of COVID became clear, assumed that from the arrival of the first cases in the UK it would probably be one or two weeks before sporadic cases and clusters occurred across the country. The influenza planning profile had been based on a worst case scenario of 50% of the population being infected with 10-12% of the local population becoming ill each week during the peak of the epidemic, following an incubation period of 1-4 days.

Depending on the virulence of the virus, the susceptibility of the population and the effectiveness of countermeasures the estimate had been that up to 2.5% of those becoming symptomatic might die, generating up to 750,000 excess deaths over and above those that may have died had a pandemic not taken place. However in the model for influenza it had been assumed that since 2009 there was little likelihood of a virus with both a high attack rate and severe disease against which medical counter-measures were ineffective and the modellers had settled on a figure of between 210,000-315,000 as a basis for the actions that might need to be taken for short term measures in an exceptional situation for additional mortuary capacity and funeral arrangements.

The local authorities are held to be the lead organisation in planning for excess deaths, working with a range of other organisations in Local Resilience Forums to involve coroners, funeral directors, mortuary managers, burial and cremation authorities in addition to faith communities in a multi-agency approach.

Preventing the NHS from falling over and the impact on death in the community
By the second and third weeks in March, with the numbers of cases and deaths doubling every two to three days, the pressure to ensure that the NHS did not fall over had been growing. This lay

behind both the creation of the Nightingale hospitals but also the discharge of large numbers of hospital patients to care homes.

It also led to the adoption of a policy to reduce the numbers of frail elderly and others suffering with long term conditions being admitted to hospitals in the first place. Clinical teams had begun to develop clinical protocols to guide their decisions—not least with regard to determining whether or not it was appropriate to transfer patients from a domestic to a hospital setting. This began to be formalised through the triaging of those aged over 65 years. Beginning with a clinical assessment at a GP surgery, in an NHS-111 call, or via the local corona command centre, decisions had begun to be taken as to whether patients might benefit from hospital treatment taking into account other factors, including their level of frailty as assessed on the Rockwood Clinical frailty Score—a 9-point scale in which a cut-off point of 7 or more indicated severe or very severe frailty, or being terminally ill and approaching the end of life. Tools such as this and the National Institute for Health and Care Excellence (NICE), rapid guideline for critical care in adults, published on 20 March were intended to bring some objectivity into a process that in the end needed to be highly person-centred and subjective.

Almost immediately the NICE guidelines proved to be highly controversial and led to criticism and outrage as to its ethical basis and it was revised on 25 March. The initial guidance had appeared to suggest that patients with learning disabilities or with stable long term disabilities such as cerebral palsy might be assessed using a clinical frailty tool which might render them unsuitable for hospital treatment. It seemed that the imperatives of the NHS were intruding in an unacceptable way on the ethical practice of medicine.

At the same time, with the rapidly increasing numbers of COVID-19 cases and deaths—and as the potential for 'Exceedance' of critical care in hospitals loomed large, together with fear among non-COVID patients of acquiring the virus in hospital, some commentators tried to initiate a debate at a community and family level about end of life choices. Sometimes this was clumsy and had more than a eugenic edge to it and steering a sensitive and ethically grounded path was difficult.

It is known from research that whilst a majority of those nearing the end of their lives would prefer to die at home a majority of their loved ones are reluctant for this to happen from fear of being unsupported and out of their depth. This is an area of life which deserves much more attention in normal times. In the event the timely publication of a most sensitive and practical guide, 'Caring for Your Dying Relative at Home with COVID-19' by Hospice UK Vice President, Professor Baroness Finlay of LLandaff was a major contribution to this vexed question.

Funerals and all that
As the numbers of deaths escalated the planning arrangements for increasing mortuary capacity kicked in, with temporary mortuaries being established around the country.

For many families that had already been through the traumatic experience of being unable to hold the hand and share the last moments of a loved one in a hospital infectious diseases or intensive care unit, the situation they now found themselves in was a grief too far. Funerals quickly became a flash point in the war against the coronavirus with councils and funeral directors taking different approaches to limiting the number of mourners and reports of a failure to provide adequate PPE for the safe handling of bodies or the rituals of the funeral. On 22 March the *Guardian* reported that the coroner in Lancashire had taken it upon himself to give COVID-19 advice because of the lack of PPE advising funeral directors to create makeshift face masks out of 'towels, bin liners and incontinence pads'.

Fran Hall, one of the authors of *The Good Funeral Guide* spoke for many on 27 March, when she said 'with the heaviest of hearts, today we are going against everything that *The Good Funeral Guide* has become known for over the years, and calling for funerals to be stopped completely'. She went on to say that 'the decision to exempt funerals from the current ban on social gatherings was undoubtedly made for compassionate reasons but the current lack of clear instruction and direction is leading to anguish and suffering beyond imagination.... grieving people are ending up with a funeral that has been pared down to something almost unrecognisable... It's breaking people's hearts... We will probably never know the damage that it's being done to people's hearts and souls, their emotional and mental wellbeing, their ability to grieve and survive in a newly empty, frightening world'.

This situation was compounded for the angry relatives of hundreds of NHS frontline workers who had died caring for the corona sick when they learned that their loved ones would not be entitled to inquests exploring the failure of government to ensure their health and safety through regular testing of those in hospitals or the adequate provision of PPE. On 3 April Kirklees Metropolitan Council followed Bradford and Leeds in halting crematorium funeral services across the borough.

In the absence of government guidance Humanists UK had issued its own on 23 March, covering PPE and body bags; advice that there should be no open coffins, viewings or embalming, that mourners should be a maximum of 5, no pall-bearing, bibles, orders of service, flowers or touching of artefacts; but stressing the importance of short, meaningful services focussed on the committal of the body together with improvements to the infrastructure for streaming services.

On 31 March the government issued updated Guidance for Care of the Deceased with Suspected or Confirmed Coronavirus COVID-19, and funeral directors, funeral celebrants and the leaders of faith communities digested the implications for their duties and responsibilities.

The main principles underpinning official guidance were that the bodies of those who had died as a result of coronavirus and the bereaved family should be treated with sensitivity, dignity and respect and that people who work in those services, as well as mourners, should be protected from infection. Detailed instruction was provided with regard to handling bodies and the avoidance of potential aerosols, the limits on the number of permitted mourners, details of the social distancing requirements and direction on the exclusion of those from participating in funeral rituals who could be harbouring the virus. It was made explicit that mourners should not take part in rituals or practices that would bring them into close contact with the body and that contact with the body should be restricted to those who were wearing PPE and had been trained in its appropriate use. In view of the pressure on funeral services, burial and cremation, together with the requirements of the directive, there was a move to foreshortened, 'direct' funerals with the expectation that the bereaved would hold a later event to celebrate the loved ones demise.

As has been discussed earlier with regard to the challenge of infection control in particular faith communities this was also potentially an issue when it came to burial. On the issue of virus transmission before lockdown, there was more of a risk in the worshipping communities which were not part of a larger worshipping infrastructure, or eschewed the institution of which they were a part. Individual churches, mosques and places of worship found themselves exercising decision-making autonomy without engaging with professional advice. Although the Church of England and the Roman Catholic Church were able to give all institutions guidance, the Muslim Council of Britain also began to act in a more institutional way, issuing guidance on a par with institutional Christian churches. Whilst around the country these vital matters could be characterised as 'muddling through', in other places such as Liverpool, were there were well-established arrangements for collaboration, such as the Death Management Cell of the Merseyside Resilience Forum and the Faith Leaders Group in the Liverpool City region, were able to bring some coherence to a complex and potentially chaotic situation.

For the Rector of Liverpool Parish Church, Crispin Pailing, during the pandemic different faith groups found different areas for compromise; for example in death rituals the Hindu and Jewish communities found it relatively easy, although emotionally difficult, to suspend many of their rituals with dead bodies, Muslim rites were reduced, although in some form ritual washing still took place. The intensity of the situation with rapidly filling mortuaries and the need for PPE when washing bodies meant that there was unparalleled engagement with faith rituals by local government and the NHS.

Whereas both Jews and Muslims expect burial within 24 hours or so of death, on Merseyside there has long been provision for weekend burial of Jewish dead but not for Muslims. Parity of provision was achieved within an hour of the Death Management Cell becoming aware of the first death of a Muslim.

Lack of knowledge between faith communities of their respective rituals was an ongoing issue, for example with regard to the use of shrouds rather than coffins in Muslim burial, bringing with it the need for more undistanced people to lower the body into the grave. In contrast to the prompt burial requirements of Muslims and Jews the desire of cultural Christians for funerals to be celebrations of the deceased's life led to pressure for delay which was difficult to accommodate in view of body storage challenges; this necessitated a joint communications initiative by the Church of England Bishop and Roman Catholic Archbishop to take their followers with them. Some faith groups found it easier to move their ceremonies online than others and for some, despite an expressed willingness to conform to public-health guidance there were those who found ways around the restriction on numbers at funerals bringing concomitant risk of further outbreaks. The return to place based worship, with the easing of lockdown, brought with it fresh challenges with some mosques delaying opening for fears of the numbers turning up whilst some churches sought to minimise risk by promoting safer ways of social distancing in small groups after short services.

The public-health challenges posed by the visitation of a pandemic that strikes individual families out of the blue are immense and can leave behind a long trail of mental health fallout to compound the physical loss or disability. By July 4 the best estimate is that about 65,000 people had died during the pandemic in the UK although a proportion of these individual people may have been nearing the end of their natural lives, their loss is no less for those to whom they were a spouse, mother or father, brother or sister, grandfather or grandmother, or a dear friend. Many thousands of such people perished unnecessarily during the COVID 2020 pandemic in the UK because of our lack of pre-paredness and inadequate response.

'No man is an island, entire of itself;
Every man is a piece of the continent, a part of the main.
. . .
Any man's death diminishes me,
because I am involved in mankind,
And therefore never send to know for whom the bell tolls;
It tolls for thee'
John Donne, 1624

18

Independent SAGE

With the steep rise in corona cases and deaths in early April, which was to reach its peak between 8 and 10 April, the government's response began to attract increasing criticism. Boris Johnson had been admitted to hospital on 6 and after a period spent in intensive care was discharged to his country residence at Chequers for a period of convalescence. In his absence there was confusion, a sense of drift and concerns about a power vacuum at the heart of government, with Dominic Raab deputising 'where necessary' but Johnson refusing to give up the reins pending full recovery.

On 22 April a *Financial Times* analysis of data from the Office of National statistics suggested that the pandemic had already caused at least 41,000 deaths, more than double the figure of 17,337 published by the government. By this time some of the members of the Scientific Advisory Group for Emergencies (SAGE), were becoming wary that by their deflection of criticism onto their advisers by saying that they had been 'guided by the scientific and medical advice' SAGE, together with the Chief Medical Officer and Chief Scientific Adviser, were being set up as a 'Human shield' for government. Matters were not helped by the lack of transparency of the SAGE deliberations in the form of publication of minutes or even the details of the membership of its committees.

In response to a request from Greg Clark MP, chair of the

House of Commons Science and Technology Select Committee, to Sir Patrick Vallance, the chair of SAGE, for more information about the structure, membership and operational processes of SAGE, Vallance had made a formal response on 4 April. In this he identified four expert contributory groups feeding into SAGE: the Scientific Influenza Group on Modelling (40-45 participants); The Scientific Pandemic Influenza Group on Behavioural Science (18 participants); the New and Emerging Respiratory Virus Threats Advisory Group (16 participants) and the Clinical Information Network (5 participants). He described the range of backgrounds of the groups memberships as covering molecular evolution, epidemiology, clinical science and practice, modelling emerging infectious diseases, behavioural science, statistics, virology and microbiology. Other Sage participants included the Chief Medical Officer, PHE, Medical Director for NHS England, the Office of National Statistics, the NHS, the Food Standards Agency, Health and Safety Executive, and Chief Scientific Advisers of government departments relevant to specific meetings or their own scientific expertise. There was no mention of input from practising local Directors of Public Health, and little evidence of anthropological or public-health history insights.

Sir Patrick went on to defend the decision to not disclose the SAGE membership on the grounds of 'safeguarding individual members personal security and protects them from lobbying and other forms of unwanted influence which may hinder their ability to give impartial advice'. The public was no wiser about the membership of the main SAGE committee itself and no mention was made of the close relationship that Sir Patrick had enjoyed with the pharmaceutical industry.

By 23 April, according to the *Guardian*, independent experts were expressing growing frustration at the government's claim to be 'following the science' and expressing concerns that the views of public-health experts were being overlooked, with disproportionate weight being given to the views of modellers. At the beginning of the emergency only one of the four complementary territories of the UK had a Chief Medical Officer who was trained and fully qualified in public health, (Frank Atherton in Wales). Catherine Calderwood, Chief Medical Officer of Scotland, was an obstetrician and gynaecologist; Michael McBride, Chief Medical Officer for Northern Ireland, had a research background as a clinician in HIV/AIDS; and Chris Whitty, Chief Medical Officer for England, was a clinical epidemiologist in infectious diseases.

The following day the *Guardian* revealed the membership of SAGE as comprising 21 non-political advisers from a narrow range of backgrounds, together with two Downing Street political advisers, Dominic Cummings and data specialist Ben Warner, who had been at the heart of the Conservative Party successful general election campaign in December 2019 and had modelled the data for the Vote Leave Brexit campaign. Of the 21 other advisers, 14 were male, 7 female, and all but one were drawn from London, Oxford and Cambridge. The odd one out was Professor Andrew Rambaut. He was from the Institute of Environmental Biology in Edinburgh, so hardly a choice that dispelled the impression of a cosy group stuck in a mid-century time capsule.

The chair of one of the feeder groups to SAGE, Professor Graham Medley, of the London School of Hygiene and Tropical Medicine, and chair of the group on modelling, was one of the first to elaborate on the herd immunity strategy on Friday 13 March. He told Newsnight that he'd like to 'put all the more vulnerable people into the north of Scotland… everybody else into Kent and have a nice, big epidemic in Kent, so that everybody becomes immune'.

One of those who expressed concern about the membership of SAGE and its modus operandi was Sir David King who said that he was 'shocked 'to discover there were political advisers on SAGE, adding that 'if you are giving science advice, your advice should be free of any political bias' political advisers had never been on the equivalent committees of SAGE when he had chaired them during the Blair government.

On 3 May Sir David King announced that he was to set up a shadow version of the government's SAGE to counter the growing concerns about 'dangerous' political interference in advice to government. He had assembled a group of 12 independent experts, 'in response to concerns about the lack of transparency'. Included among the members were four very experienced and highly respected public-health consultants with practical experience, something which had been lacking until now.

In establishing the new group Sir David told the *Sunday Times* 'I am not critical of the scientists who are putting advice before the Government... but because there is no transparency, the government can say they are following scientific advice but we don't know they are'. This move finally prompted the chair of SAGE, Patrick Vallance, to announce that he would publish a partial list of the official government advisers and begin to publish minutes of meetings, albeit sometimes heavily redacted.

Following a press conference the next day the new independent body published the first of a series of reports the following week on May 12, attracting a great deal of interest and a metaphorical sigh of relief from a welcoming public. This first Independent SAGE Report, 'COVID-19: what are the options for the UK?', reviewed the current state of knowledge about the pandemic and identified the key issues that needed to be addressed to re-establish trust in the government response and in securing effective action. The report identified the priorities for action to support the gradual release from social distancing by means of a sustainable response, until such a time as effective treatments or vaccines became available. The authors of the report chose not to focus on the structural and procedural weaknesses that had contributed to the UK's dire failure to measure up to the response of other

215

countries of similar size and demographics, rather leaving these matters for the judicial enquiry that must inevitably follow sometime in the future.

The many criticisms of the government response to the greatest public-health emergency in a hundred years had identified the impact of ten years of austerity on the resilience of health and social care made worse by a chaotic reorganisation in 2013 and the establishment of a highly centralising national public-health agency, PHE. This had been compounded by a failure to learn the lessons of poor emergency preparedness that came out of Operation Cygnus in 2016 and for the prime minister to get a grip of the parameters of the crisis early in February with a cascade of consequences. These especially involved the failure to mobilise and procure adequate capacity for coronavirus testing, for Personal Protective Equipment and for preparing the public for eventualities that subsequently became inevitable, not least the wholesale national lockdown and grinding to a halt of the economy. From early on in the government press conferences the SAGE had been pushed into the foreground behind a mantra of 'following the science' without exactly which science was being alluded to in the absence of transparency. Over time arcane, mysterious and contradictory statements and statistics had come to be clouded in a fog of poor communication.

As put by professor Brian Cox, 'There's no such thing as "the science", which is a key lesson. If you hear a politician say we're following the science, then what that means is that they don't know what science is. There isn't such a thing as "the science". Science is a mindset'. Scientific literacy was rare among senior politicians; the prime minister had a degree in classics and health minister Hancock a degree in politics, philosophy and economics, a well-trodden path for British career politicians. In a political world still dominated by C.P. Snow's 'Two Cultures' good public-health governance requires arrangements in which there is effective mutual challenge and respectful listening between politicians and the right range of advisers. What we were left with in 2020 was a form of the Emperor's new clothes in which politicians believing their own rhetoric wrapped it up in a cloak of mumbo jumbo quasi-scientific deference, whilst a narrow range of advisers, perhaps seduced by the hubris of proximity to power and the prospect of civic honours, failed to do justice to their crafts.

In contrast to the official SAGE committee with its undue deference to a dogmatic political agenda of neglect, dominated by a narrowly drawn group of Home Counties and 'golden triangle' academics, the Independent SAGE, included a suite of highly experienced and practically minded public-health consultants together with credible and complementary colleagues. Their offering, borne of the heat of a failing battle against the virus, is reminiscent in its comprehensive overview, of the 1942 Beveridge Report, that provided the blueprint for the welfare state after World War II.

The eighteen recommendations of the panel report tackle head-on the bizarre interlude of 'herd immunity'. Backing the goal of 'suppression' rather than managed spread. As repeated frequently by the Director General of WHO as well, it was essential to build the capacity to identify, isolate, test and treat, trace and quarantine all those infected with a standard 14 days isolation rather than the 7 days that had somehow slipped in from left field.

According to the Independent SAGE, real-time quality data, conforming to national data standards was essential to inform a wide range of modelling approaches. Proper attention needed to be paid to the development of whole population, safe habit formation with regard to hygiene and bio-security with reference to the range of potentially vulnerable groups and settings, including care homes, prisons, other closed institutions, ports, dis-advantaged and BAME communities. They recommended that arrangements should be made to take over hotels and other suitable places for isolation and quarantine purposes in support of these interventions and during any easing of the lockdown.

Other important issues identified were the reform of the procurement processes, to ensure that all children had personal access to technology and computing facilities in support of their continued education as a human right, strengthening health and social care planning with the provision of adequate bed numbers to ensure resilience, and the recognition of the complex and emerging clinical patterns of disease caused by the virus, including multi-system and organ damage requiring extensive after-care and rehabilitation.

In the medium and longer-term, and with a clear eye to the legacy of the ongoing public-health disaster, Sir David's team called for:

* A strengthening of the social safety net for a range of groups including older people, those on low income, BAME groups; the proper co-ordination of emergency preparedness and response across government at national, devolved administration and local government areas;
* The building up of a long term integrated and sustainable public-health infrastructure, rooted in the community in contrast to the current top-down approach;
* And the establishment of an integrated National Health and Social Care System for England.

In the midst of the chaos, the Independent SAGE was providing a glimpse of a brighter future that might be possible given the vision and political will.

19

Cummingsgate and After

If February had been a lost month, and the week beginning 9 March a critical one, then the weekend of 23 May was a tipping point of sorts. The news that Dominic Cummings, had been caught breaching the government's own rules on lockdown by travelling to his parent's house in Durham, outraged the nation and shredded what was left of trust in those leading the response to COVID-19.

The impact of the UK epidemic on NHS hospitals had begun to peak in mid-April but the parallel outbreak in care homes was escalating behind it. As the row over the obfuscation of numbers continued there was growing public awareness of the scandalous neglect of thousands of the most vulnerable and of the growing toll of deaths. On 19 May the *Guardian* revealed that temporary care home workers had transmitted COVID-19 between premises as cases surged, unmasking ministers' claims to have 'thrown a protective ring around care homes'. By then an estimated 22,000 people were believed to have died from COVID-19 related illness in these settings and on 29 of the month an adjustment to the official total number of deaths raised the overall tally from 21,749 to 26,711. These were still well below the estimates of the *Economist* or of those epidemiologists who had started making comparisons with the excess deaths from all causes over each of the previous five years.

Throughout May the chaotic and ineffective government response to the emergency was becoming more obvious with a steady spate of stories of incompetence, overpromising and under-delivering. The erosion of trust resulting from mixed messages and poor leadership was beginning to manifest itself in a breakdown of adherence to travel restrictions, mixing and social distancing. This became increasingly apparent with the special bank holiday on 8 May to mark the 75 anniversary of VE Day, when beaches, country parks and beauty spots across England were busy as people ventured further afield. Despite pleas from local authorities and public-health advisers tourist hotspots and routes to the coast were becoming very congested with the police caught in the middle of increasing confusion about what was permitted.

On 15 May, transport secretary Grant Shapps was reported as trailing yet another false dawn, this time an antibody test that would be a 'game changer'. 'I think it's very exciting that there's a very, very reliable, possibly even 100% reliable antibody test 'he said; a prospect endorsed by deputy Chief Medical Officer Jonathan Van Tam who said that the new Roche test would be 'rapidly rolled out as soon as it is possible to do so', adding that 'I think it will be incredibly important as the days, weeks, months go by' although admitting that it was still not known whether contracting the virus would give people immunity, and if so for how long.

At the same time the much vaunted NHS App, intended to transform testing and tracing, that was being tested on the Isle of Wight, was running into trouble. A split was emerging between government advisers as to whether it should be abandoned in favour of one being developed by Apple and Google that posed fewer ethical issues of confidentiality and seemed more likely to be both acceptable to the public and to actually work. And on the same day it was revealed that the government had spent £20 million on HIV and anti-malarial drugs that had been heavily promoted by President Trump despite scepticism from experienced infectious disease physicians; in addition published research in the *New England Journal of Medicine* concluded that the anti-virals Lopanivir and Ritonavir 'did not show any observable benefit'.

Meanwhile: a belated effort to recruit thousands of contact tracers as part of a central initiative to test and trace appeared to be in trouble with reports of rushed and chaotic recruitment and superficial training for what was in essence a sophisticated role requiring well a developed personal skill set; at the same time the symptoms of loss of taste and smell, although a recurring theme from the clinical front line only now made it into clinical diagnostic protocols with the suggestion that tens of thousands of cases of COVID-19 may have been missed because of the failure to alert the public to this early manifestation of infection.

Amid reports that keeping schools closed was almost certainly increasing educational inequalities between the wealthiest and poorest children a new fault line opened up with a row about whether it was safe for the nation's state schools to reopen before the end of the summer term, by and large the private school sector having opted to wait until September. Into this toxic mix the newspapers began to report that at the height of the pandemic and lockdown the Cummings family had made their escape from London to Durham and Barnard Castle with Dominic Cummings having tested positive for the virus.

Travelling to Durham and eye testing in Barnard Castle
Over the weekend of 23/24 May the story broke in the *Guardian* and the Daily Mirror of Dominic Cummings visit to Durham after he had been seen rushing out of Downing Street the day the prime minister tested positive for the virus on 27 March. Cummings had

developed symptoms of COVID over the next two days and his explanation was that the family had travelled to his parent's house where they would be able to take advantage of family support for their small son while Cummings was ill. It later transpired that not only had he and his family travelled the 264 miles north but in addition he and his wife had visited Barnard Castle, some 16 miles from Durham, on his wife's birthday. This was ostensibly to test whether his eyesight was good enough to drive back to London his having experienced optical symptoms from the viral infection not previously reported by other sufferers. The reason why his driver wife could not have driven back to London was never explained. In addition his wife, Mary Wakefield, had been posting misleading information on social media sites implying that the family were spending the entire lockdown in London.

This episode coincided with the resignation of epidemic modeller Professor Neil Ferguson because of his having received a home visit from his girlfriend during lockdown and the resignation of the Chief Medical Officer for Scotland, Catherine Calderwood, because of the visits she had made with her family to their weekend cottage outside Edinburgh. The allegations of hypocrisy hung heavily in the air.

Over the next week the political pressure grew on Dominic Cummings and on the prime minister with calls for Cummings to resign. It appeared that after he had been seen in Durham by retired chemistry teacher, Robin Lees, who reported him to the police, he had received a visit from a member of the Durham Constabulary who gave him advice but took no further action. With front-page headlines every day for the next week Cummings was in no mood to apologise, telling the *Guardian* 'I don't regret what I did 'and refusing calls to resign despite a clamour from Conservative MPs. In a press conference, held, uniquely for a non-elected government adviser, in the rose garden at 10 Downing Street, Cummings failed to answer fundamental questions as to why he should have broken a lockdown that applied to everybody else.

The prime minister brushed aside a revolt by almost 100 of his own members of Parliament saying that he regarded the matter as closed and forbidding the Chief Medical Officer, Professor Chris Whitty and Chief Scientific Adviser, Patrick Vallance, from commenting on the matter in the daily press conference. This gagging of Johnson's most senior scientific advisers, marked a watershed in both public perceptions of the cosy relationship between advisers and politicians and was also the moment after which health professionals began to break ranks from a position of solidarity with the government. When asked about Cummings and the lockdown in one of the press conferences at the end of the week, Deputy Chief Medical Officer Jonathan Van Tam said that the lockdown rules 'are clear and they have always been clear. In my opinion they are for the benefit of all. In my opinion they apply to all'. He was not to appear again at a press conference for some days. It would later transpire that the government's Chief Nursing Officer Ruth May had been stood down from a press conference when she refused to toe the line about Cummings.

With the story still running after over a week the *Observer* reported on 31 May that Britain's top public-health leaders and scientists had warned Johnson in a letter that trust in the government had been shattered by the Dominic Cummings affair and that it would pose a real danger to life once lockdown measures began to be lifted later that week.

They went on to warn that there had been a failure to set up an effective test trace and isolate system to identify and quarantine newly infected people and that as a result they were 'very concerned for the safety and wellbeing of the general public'. Until this point the medical establishment had mostly held its counsel whilst the government prevaricated, doing too little too late and being highly selective in its choice of evidence to make decisions. The public-health establishment had also sat on its hands unwilling to criticise either PHE in its failings and lack of visibility, the limp behaviour of the government advisers or the government's incompetence; many of its senior voices had been compromised in their endorsement of the unsupportable and local Directors of Public health had been explicitly gagged. This now began to change.

Lockdown too late, easing lockdown too soon
If the government had been slow to act at the beginning of the emergency and had then been inconsistent in its response, doing too little too late, and seeking to deflect the responsibility for difficult decisions onto others, there now began an erratic process that would lead to an ending to the lockdown. With the economic costs of the failure to get a grip on the epidemic the devastating impact to the economy was becoming daily more apparent alongside the dreadful toll of deaths. In denial of the reality that investment in public health was a prerequisite for the revival of the economy, apologists once again began to argue that there had been an over-reaction and that re-opening the economy should take precedence over public health. On 1 June the Association of Directors of Public Health put its head above the parapets to warn the government about easing off the lockdown.

Despite this and other warning voices, throughout June there was a helter skelter of announcements and initiatives increasingly pointing the way to a desire to restore 'business as usual'. Whilst the UK excess death toll passed 50,000 the head of the UK Statistics Authority accused the government of continuing to mislead the public about the number of tests being carried out for COVID-19. In a letter to Matt Hancock, Sir David Norgrove observed that 'The aim seems to be to show the largest possible number of tests, even at the expense of understanding'. The government was mixing up tests actually carried out with testing kits sent out in the post, irrespective of whether they were received, used appropriately, returned and producing a valid test result. 'this distinction is too often elided during the presentation at the daily press conference, where the relevant figure may mis-leadingly be described simply as the number of tests carried out. There are no data on how many of the tests posted out are in fact then completed successfully'.

At the same time, and a sign of the increasing number of advisers belatedly distancing themselves from the handling of the affair, Neil Ferguson was quoted as saying that he was shocked at how poorly care homes had been protected from the virus and that infections in UK care homes were now feeding into the epidemic in the wider community. Ferguson was later to go on the record as saying that had the lockdown been introduced a week earlier the number of coronavirus deaths could have been halved. Leader of the Opposition, Keir Starmer, having initially been gentle with the government, was now telling Johnson to 'Get a grip or risk a second wave of coronavirus'; and on 5 June the *Guardian* broke the news that Tony Presteigne, chief operating officer of the NHS Test and Trace system had admitted in a staff webinar that the programme would be 'imperfect' and that it would not be fully operational until September.

The *Observer* on 7 June reported that senior voices from the world of medicine including many of the Medical Royal Colleges, voices, that had been silent for so long, were pleading for the prime minister to ditch 'cheap political rhetoric' and plan for a second wave of infection. By this time too there was growing concern over the impact the epidemic had been having on BAME staff employed within the NHS, deaths of this group having accounted for a disproportionate number of the now hundreds of NHS staff deaths. By mid-June this concern had merged with the international movement 'Black Lives matter', following the killing of George Floyd by police officers in Minnesota. Despite all warnings the government was preparing the ground to let go of control.

Commenting on the UK government handling of the COVID emergency in June, among a plethora of announcements, Tony Blair said he was confused about what the rules were and were not. Interviewed by the *Sunday Times* he commented 'the government has announced a confusing array of three 'phases', three 'steps', five 'tests' and five 'alert levels'. These overlap with one another substantially, are poorly defined and assessed in opaque ways, and are not linked explicitly to the lifting of different restrictions. This opacity leaves the impression that considerations other than risk are governing the pace of easing. This lies at the root of the trust problem'. In their place Blair proposed two metrics, the 'R' rate and the number of new daily cases. Adding that thresholds could then be set for easing of lockdown measures (as was happening in Germany), but that this approach would require mass testing on a scale that had not been contemplated in the UK. A necessary refinement of Blair's proposal would have required the use of different 'R' numbers for different populations, areas and settings.

Of the various test regimes alluded to by Tony Blair, that proposed by the government after the lockdown was announced in March may seem one of the most pragmatic. The five points covered

* The ability to protect the NHS and its capacity to cope
* A sustained fall in deaths
* A falling infection rate
* Dealing with the challenges of testing and PPE
* Ensuring that there was no second peak that could overwhelm the NHS

It is noticeable that this list carried no mention of care homes or the burden of care and of deaths at home, both issues that interacted with the ability of the NHS to cope without seeming to fall over. The continuing failure to scale up testing and tracing together with a systematic failure to assure isolation of those potentially harbouring the virus potentially compromised each of the other tests and problems of PPE rumbled on into the summer.

The detail of the testing and tracing regime was itself elaborated into yet a further evaluative framework of the so-called 5 pillars, covering:

Pillar 1
Scaling up of NHS swab testing for those with a medical need and where possible the most critical key workers; this turned out to be by far the most successful part of the effort, under the control and direction of the NHS in partnership with PHE.
Pillar 2
Testing for the wider population—sub-contracted to for-profit accountancy firm Deloitte—which had been disastrous, with logistical failures involving the tests themselves, their reliability and reporting and the sharing of incomplete data with local public-health teams. As of July 6 government data showed that only 39,382 tests had been carried out against a much heralded capacity for many times this. This was only slightly more than the Pillar 1 testing for the same day, even though population level testing needed to be much higher. The Pillar 2 testing had been declining every day since 2 July when it was reported as 168,921. This was a serious failing and prevented any meaningful surveillance of rises in and distribution of infection. It was at this level that intelligence was most needed and the failure of it that led to the myriad of local outbreaks that began to manifest themselves at the beginning of July, beginning with those in slaughterhouses, meat processing factories, rag trade sweat shops in Leicester and the A.S. Green vegetable farm in Herefordshire, supplying Aldi, Asda, M&S and Sainsbury's.

Data hoarding by PHE had kept local public-health directors in the dark only to be followed by the government riding roughshod over local political and public-health leaders with the imposition of a local lockdown from London. This lack of granular data covering postcodes, ethnicity and other neighbourhood level intelligence was what prevented local public health, health-and-safety and trading standards personnel from honing in on dysfunctional cottage industry textile operations in Leicester- with exploitation of the workforce in conditions tailor made for incubating the virus.

Pillars 3 and 4

They related to mass antibody testing and population surveillance and it was very difficult to know where things had got to in view of the contradictory messages about antibody testing and the paucity of transparency information.

Pillar 5

Or the 'spearheading of a diagnostic national effort to build a mass testing capacity at a completely new scale'. Apart from the fact that only one of the five pillars had been achieved going into July, the government seemed hell bent on easing the lockdown before it was possible to be confident that the prime Minister's 'sombrero' had been well and truly squashed pending any resurgence later in the year.

It was the lack of progress on the fifth pillar that was perhaps of greatest concern. Many private sector contracts for COVID-19 work had been let outside of normal contracting governance frameworks. They had also been let to inappropriate contractors such as for PPE to a family run recruitment firm, a sweets manufacturer and a specialist in pest control products. Nevertheless the government made known its intention of awarding contracts worth £5 billion for testing to private contractors, equivalent to the entire annual spend on English NHS laboratories. The performance issues with the Pillar 2 testing hardly justified such a bonanza for the private sector given its poor performance in delivering against procurement requirements and the opportunity cost of not using this resource to rebuild much needed resilience in local public-health capacity and capability

The news of this proposed private sector commission coincided with the revelation that it was planning to renege on its agreement with NHS chief executive Simon Stevens, to provide £10 billion to cover the NHS COVID-19 overspend. The collateral damage of the COVID emergency in terms of its impact on other NHS activity, not least for patients with cancer and other conditions requiring urgent treatment and care was leading to the build-up of significant waiting lists. Without the additional monies this backlog of work was likely to give a significant boost to the private sector for those who could afford it, and long waits for with adverse health consequences for those who couldn't.

An indecent rush for the exit
Most of June was marked by efforts by government to create the impression that the crisis was coming to an end and that it was time to reboot the economy. If only No 10 had sewn up its communications about COVID in January and February with as much clarity and creativity then. No 10's freshly installed PR team, however, had a task that had little to do with informing the public: save the skin of No 10, blame others. Thus, having managed to put Cummingsgate behind him, the prime minister now began to distance himself from his scientific advisers with increasing indications that it would be they together with an anonymous PHE and its senior professionals, Simon Stevens, the Chief Executive of the NHS, and even the British public who could now be blamed for ignoring the lockdown and social distancing, and so would be blamed for the country's appalling showing in the face of COVID-19. The hand of Dominic Cummings in the spate of diversionary announcements and initiatives was not far.

Meanwhile the Downing Street press conferences to inform the public were watered down and then discontinued, further confusing and obfuscatory changes were made to the timings and framing of published COVID statistics and it was announced that in future the government would adopt the US model of having a public-relations professional appearing before the media to answer questions. As the devolved governments of Scotland, Wales and Northern Ireland, that had hung together for the first months of the emergency with the London administration, went their own ways, they increasingly demonstrated more grip and an ability to aim for zero cases in their own territories. However the more isolated the Johnson cabinet ended up being, the more grandiose its claims became.

Among the chaos and confusion there was good news from the researchers who had demonstrated that the cheap and longstanding pharmaceutical dexamethasone might have a role to play in reducing the severity of the illness in a proportion of patients. However conflicting evidence was being reported on the potential benefits of vitamin D and great uncertainty about benefits to be had from other pharmaceutical treatments or the prospects for reliable antibody tests and for effective vaccines in the near future. Increasingly it began to look as if the world would have to live with COVID-19 and adapt the way we live rather than hoping for science to provide a magic bullet.

The indecent rush to a premature exit from lockdown before robust arrangements were in place for mass testing and tracing together with assurance of compliance with self-isolation and quarantine resulted in a chaotic period of announcements and controversies leading up to 4 July, the end of Britain's enforced lockdown. Prominent among these was the declared intention to re-open the state primary schools for three year groups: reception, year 1 and year 6, despite warnings from independent scientists that it was too early to re-open while transmission and infection rates remained so high.

While most of England's primary schools were set to open from June 1, a large majority of teachers said that they would not be able to accommodate all three year groups in the necessary reduced class sizes to conform to the necessary social distancing and biosecurity. The move was highly controversial with parents and on the appointed day an estimated one million children were kept home. Later in the month the government decided to abandon the requirement for reduced class sizes, insisting that from September the schools would be back to normal. Concerns expressed by the Children's Commissioner, Anne Longfield, about the impact of the epidemic on children's mental and physical health and the need for remedial action passed without response.

Having failed to act on active measures to screen, test, trace and isolate where necessary, travellers entering the country from early on the Home Secretary, Priti Patel, took it on herself to do too much too late. On May 22 she had announced that nearly all international arrivals at UK ports, including air, sea and rail, would have to quarantine for 14 days from June 8. Having failed to prevent people entering from high prevalence areas such as Italy and Austria when the pandemic was seeding into the country, it now seemed that the country with one of the highest rates of infection was intent on penalising travellers from countries whose prompt actions had led to them now having low levels of infection. The response was uproar from the travel industry and as the controversy reverberated through the month the decision was eventually taken to relax the requirements.

Rising concern about the economy with dire predictions of accumulating debt and dramatic increases in unemployment rates after the government furlough scheme came to an end were understandable. At the same time the confusion over the messages coming from government as to what was and was not permitted led to a rapid erosion of compliance with the social distancing that had been so important in driving down infection rates. Whilst the epidemic curve of deaths declined sharply during late May and early June it then flattened off and continued to run at between 100-200 reported daily deaths into July; this was in marked contrast to those countries whose preparedness and response had enabled them to drive infections down with the realistic goal of zero further infections before the end of the summer.

The breakdown in personal discipline and adherence to social distancing was one widely manifested. At weekends and during the may bank holidays there had been worryingly scenes of large numbers of people crowding open spaces, beaches and parks with little respect for the two metre rule of personal space. This was now further confused by reports that the government was intent on reducing the two metres to one metre and continuing confusion about whether the wearing of masks was either recommended or required. In due course the issue of mask wearing would lead to even more confusion in early July with ministers giving contradictory messages about the requirement to use of masks on public transport, shops and offices and other public places and minister Michael Gove being photographed in Pret-A-Manger without a mask.

One of the most dramatic examples of the breakdown in compliance concerning social gatherings followed Liverpool FC finally securing the 2019-20 Premier League Championship when Chelsea beat Manchester City 2-1 at Stamford Bridge. It was always going to be a problematic moment but the worst fears were realised over the next few nights with huge crowds celebrating around Liverpool's Anfield ground and at the Pierhead. A desperate Liverpool manager, Jurgen Klopp together with local Public Health Director, Matthew Ashton, appealed to the public to celebrate at home but it was too late to prevent a local spike in new confirmed infections over the next two weeks. This was followed by a further outbreak in South Liverpool following the congregation of large numbers of youths drinking on the street following the re-opening of bars in Woolton Village.

While traditional recreational establishments such as restaurants and clubs began to go out of business at a steady rate, there were reports of a revival of spontaneous 'Raves' taking place at short notice and publicised on social media, usually on fields or woodland adjacent to urban areas, posing public order challenges to the police and a not inconsiderable problem of litter.

As the country moved towards 4 July, Johnson encouraged the public to go out and shop. Having repeatedly pretended to be Winston Churchill, the man who had fought tirelessly for liberty, Johnson now moved on to channelling Franklin D. Roosevelt, the US president who had delivered his country from The Depression rather than pushed his country's worst recession on record. Johnson announced his 'New Deal' of economic measures to get the country moving again after 4 July with great pomp. The deal added up to Johnson bringing forward £5 billion of spending according to Channel 4's award-winning fact-checkers.

As the general sense that the epidemic was on the way out grew, whipped up by government messaging and despite evidence to the contrary, the *Daily Express* carried a front page photograph of Johnson pulling a pint of beer in a pub to the headline 'Cheers Boris! Here's To a Brighter Future' and all day drinking was encouraged at the nation's pubs and bars with many scheduled to open at 6 am on July 4. In the event, although the media carried coverage of large crowds in Soho and some other traditional entertainment areas, the footfall on the nation's high streets was less than had been feared with the incitement to 'Shop, Shop, Shop' falling on many deaf ears to the concern of traditional retail establishments.

July 4 came and went and was followed by a flurry of further announcements that might help the economy get back on its feet including incitement from the prime minister for people to stop home working if possible and go back to their offices and workplaces. The indications were that a significant proportion of the population that had a choice, had other ideas and were rethinking their lifestyles, work-life balance, where they wished to live and bring up their children, and whether they wished to return to the rat race of 9-5 work and lengthy commutes. There was little sign that the British government was embracing the opportunity presented by the crisis to reshape the economy and take advantage of a potential bonus of sustainability and increased public wellbeing.

The rush to return to 'business as usual' was also the focus of the reports from independent SAGE, whose fresh thinking was in marked contrast to the narrow, inhibited and belated reflections of the government's own SAGE.

From early on, once the enormity of what was facing the country began to be evident, government ministers had been constantly revising the narrative of what had been happening and the errors that were still being made; 'backfilling the truth' as it was being described. A theme of the whole management of the pandemic had been a reluctance by Johnson to take charge, rather than outsourcing decisions to others and shielding himself from any accruing blame. This was becoming more explicit with criticism of the NHS, PHE and the prime minister's advisers themselves. Increasingly those advisers had been briefing their own revised narratives, getting their retaliation in first, in advance of any future enquiry and putting the best gloss on their own omissions, commissions and failure to speak truth to power.

On 16 July, the Chief Scientific Adviser, Patrick Vallance, took the opportunity of an appearance before the Science and Technology Committee to reframe his own contributions, disagreeing with the prime minister's call for people to stop home working, claiming that he had been a supporter of face masks all along and that he had been recommending the lock down since the 16 of March when many thousands of lives would have been saved; he made no reference to the many other controversial decisions and recommendations that had been made by the committee he chaired including his raising of 'herd immunity' in the week of March 9 that had caused such confusion and concern.

In the *Daily Mail* of 17 July the Chief Medical Officer was quoted as being 'very uneasy 'about moves to ease social distancing rules'. It was very difficult to imagine either Sir Donald Acheson or Sir Liam Donaldson, two of his most distinguished predecessors, pulling their punches so limply.

In many ways the advent of Independent SAGE had been a game changer in showing up the lack of fitness for purpose of the official scientific advisory committee. Its series of online meetings and reports had brought a freshness and transparency to the questions and evidence base that both the public, the professionals and the media was desperate for. In its seventh report, 'A Better Way To Go: Towards a Zero COVID UK', the committee made 7 key points and proposed 5 planks for a forward strategy to deal with the pandemic:

7 Key Points
* The prospect of many thousands of further deaths from COVID-19 over the next nine months is unacceptable
* The UK government must propose and share with the public a strategic plan on how the pandemic is going to be managed in the next 12 months and of how the various measures against the pandemic fit together in an integrated plan
* Independent SAGE believes that this strategy should have as its prime objective the achievement of a Zero COVID Britain and Ireland
* It will require the government in Whitehall to replace their failing NHS Test and Trace System with a fully-fledged and

locally controlled system of Find, Test, Trace, Isolate, Support (FTTIS)

* The Republic of Ireland, Scotland and Northern Ireland already have fewer deaths and very small numbers of new positive cases. They have the virus under control and are well placed to achieve the elimination of the virus.

* England and Wales will need to make the necessary efforts as soon as possible to achieve the same position

* Achieving elimination would allow all social distancing measures to be lifted, schools to be fully open, the hospitality and entertainment industries to reopen fully, revitalisation of the economy and a sense of much needed normality for the population.

Arguing that the UK must fundamentally change its approach Independent SAGE proposed that the strategic planks for achieving Zero COVID-19 UK should be to:

* Fully develop community-based and locally led Find, Test, Trace, Isolate and Support (FTTIS) programmes with expanded local laboratory provision, involvement of local public sector organisations and provision of all the resources necessary to enable adherence to the regulations on notification of infectious disease

* Restrict loosening of lockdown measures in any part of the UK until control of the outbreak has been achieved in that country

* Put in place well designed and scientifically based plans to act swiftly to localise, contain and suppress completely flare-ups in COVID-19 infections.

* Restrict incoming or outgoing personal travel internationally and within Britain and Ireland to the extent necessary to maintain control of the epidemic and, in particular to ensure

effective isolation of incoming passengers

* Combine all these measures with a systematic public information campaign stressing that things are not 'back to normal' yet, that premature removal of restrictions in the midst of a deadly pandemic threatens to squander all the sacrifices of lockdown and that strict compliance with restrictions now will make a full return to normality come sooner.

It was no surprise to find that this measured and evidence based approach would soon be met by politically motivated trolling and efforts to undermine the credibility of the highly able and grounded Independent SAGE committee.

Afterword

The charge sheet was long in August and stretched back to include many from previous governments. As with most major disasters there was in retrospect a terrible inevitability about it. Public health and prevention had played second fiddle to hospital medicine for decades. Years of austerity had had a huge impact on the resilience of the NHS and the fragmentation and incoherence of the 2012 Health and Social Care Act had weakened both the NHS and the public health system still further.

All this had been exacerbated by the UK's response being based on a narrow reference group of advisers, flaky data and questionable modelling. The government's approach seemed to have been to look around the world at what was working elsewhere in practice and to dismiss it as not working in theory. This had been combined with a hopeless communications function from an inadequate and over-centralised PHE.

Apportioning blame in such a comprehensive mess was going to be difficult and the immediate challenge was still to cope with the potentially impending second wave of the epidemic. The first wave of COVID attacked mainly the adult population, but it was a possibility that the second-wave spread of the virus would reach Britain's school children and could lead to deaths there. Nevertheless lessons had to be learned and the responsibilities for the first wave be placed squarely on the shoulders of those leaders who let the public down so badly, beginning with prime minister Boris Johnson.

What was attempted by the prime minister and his cabinet was to get away with what Engels described as the 'social murder' of tens of thousands of UK citizens who perished unnecessarily, removed from relatives, in our hospitals, care homes, prisons and homes during the first wave of the pandemic.

Scapegoats were lined up in the form of SAGE, individual advisers, civil servants, the Chief Executive of the NHS, Simon Stevens, frontline staff in hospitals and care homes, disposable ministers including the health secretary Matt Hancock, and most recently the general public for not doing what they were told, however incoherently. As the focus shifts to local outbreaks, local authorities and local public-health teams will be next in line.

The axe fell first over PHE, an obvious move in view of PHE's abysmal performance on a close par to the cabinet's. But it was one which was to distract attention from the assignment of political responsibility and the need for fundamental reform, strengthening and decentralisation of public health in England and Wales. Curbing the powers of NHS England and the establishment of a national Joint Biosecurity Centre should be seen in the same light—as distracting tactics that risk further dysfunctional central-isation when the need for decentralisation of power, structures, functions and resources is one of the central lessons of the crisis.

Starting with the framing of the current crisis. The clue was in the declaration of COVID-19 becoming a 'Public Health Emergency of International Concern' on 30 January. This was not primarily a hospital emergency, only becoming one when public-health systems failed. In the UK the primary responsibility for dealing with a public-health emergency lies with the public-health system in England and its equivalent bodies in Scotland, Wales and Northern Ireland. In practice PHE set the agenda as the senior partner until a parting of the ways by the devolved governments well into the pandemic.

The cross-cutting nature of public health was such that an

agency such as PHE did not have direct control over many of the issues that need to be addressed to protect health. As at the local level, the role of the central public-health system is to convene, facilitate and assure itself and government that those issues are being dealt with; for example education and employment, wider communications and cultural and sporting matters, transport, agriculture and food as well as the NHS.

It was for this reason that the departmental link of PHE to the Department of Health, dominated as it is by the NHS and hospitals agenda, is flawed. The appropriate relationship would be to the Cabinet Office with its own Minister located there with direct access across all government departments. It was also the reason why it was not appropriate to look to a Chief Medical Officer not trained in public health, to head up the public-health advice to government. The logical arrangement would be to have a fully-trained public-health professional as a National Advisor of Public Health also based in the Cabinet Office. Similarly at the local level, the position of Local Director of Public Health should by statute be required to be a board level position in each unitary local authority.

This was not to say that an agency such as PHE or its successor did not have direct responsibilities. In relationship to the COVID pandemic those responsibilities included oversight of the relevant data sets for notification of cases of the disease and deaths from it, and ensuring that the necessary intelligence was readily available to public-health teams and partners at each level to enable them to intervene. In the current crisis the charge against PHE was that it failed in this duty through over-centralisation, by not ensuring comprehensive and high quality intelligence and through data hoarding, creating a Chinese wall at the centre. Similarly the responsibility of PHE to assure the provision of adequate case finding, testing, tracing and isolating and the provision of adequate PPE for all those government staff who needed it, must be seen as an overarching assurance function of health protection that should fall to the public health system. That it failed in these duties created a major challenge and potential crisis for the NHS and especially the hospital sector.

Despite the prime minister's singling out Simon Stevens and NHS England for blame, the NHS had so far done a remarkable job under difficult circumstances. That the hospital service didn't 'fall over' in the first wave of the pandemic was as a result of some remarkably adept adaptation in a very short time. Criticism of the decision to discharge patients to care homes to free up beds and the construction of the Nightingale hospitals in fourteen days which were never used, should be seen in the light of the government and PHE's failure to get to grips with the UK epidemic in February and March. This brought huge pressure to bear on hospitals that could have been partly avoided and led to drastic measures being taken. The failure to develop testing and tracing at scale and to procure adequate PPE led directly to the spread of infections within and outside hospitals and probably played an important role in igniting the parallel epidemic in care homes. The NHS was the governmental backstop that delivered on capacity under complex circumstances.

Notwithstanding the failings of government advisers to truly speak truth to power, of agencies to fulfil their responsibilities, and of professional bodies in sitting on their hands in the early weeks of the emergency, the opportunistic use of the complexity of government by Johnson, Cummings and the cabinet, to pretend it wasn't them who controlled the levers of Whitehall was breath-taking. By the use of rapid changes of subject, dead cats, sleights of hand and diversionary tactics they drew headlines away from public-health realities and the challenges ahead. The pursuit of 'business as usual' was a chimera that would potentially lead us down a cul-de-sac of a dreadful second wave and throw away the opportunity of re-engineering our economy and a way of life to be safer, fairer and more sustainable for the whole of Britain's population.

We had to fundamentally review and transform our social and economic lives as well as the physical environments of our towns and cities if our economy is to thrive and compete with others in the new normal that will be the future. 'Business as usual' would not be that future. Johnson's empty rhetoric needed to be exposed for what it was. The key choices and errors were all political. Responsibility for them rests with the prime minister. In the British system institutions will take you where you want to go if you take the wheel and drive them. Being an absentee to invisible prime minister was the reason and not the excuse for his mismanagement. For much of the time, with a part-time, narcissistic and distracted Johnson, nobody had been at the wheel. This was not primarily the responsibility of the institutions, but nor were they exonerated by it.

The main failures of leadership seem to have come from a combination of English exceptionalism, inexperience, the misplaced application of a 'Take Back Control' campaigning approach to communications together with a lack of grip, competence, imagination and empathy. The UK government had plenty of models to follow, and the advantage at the beginning of a lag time to learn from. It was increasingly clear why others were more successful. Again and again, from South Korea, Vietnam and Taiwan, Bahrain, to Greece, Germany, Ireland, Scotland and the Isle of Mann, Ceredigion, Groningen, better outcomes have followed from obviously better leadership. Their leaders cared to engage and go the extra mile.

The prime minister and those around him in the cabinet were confident of getting away with their appalling crime of social killing, relying on things eventually coming good and public memory moving on. They controlled Parliament, the Executive and the flows of information to the media. Most of the mainstream media tended to be compliant and the opposition pulled its punches. There were few signs of systematic, sustained and politically thought-through challenge. We could all do better than this.

One of the most positive recent developments was the establishment of the Independent SAGE by Sir David King. This quickly became a trusted source of analysis and advice that was clearly acting in the public interest rather than in the interests of a few men in Downing Street. Surely the time had come for Independent SAGE to launch its own Independent Interim Enquiry to establish key scientific and other issues in a rigorous, independent and focused way. Its conclusions would provide a point of reference for the eventual official enquiry, forcing the burden of proof onto the prime minister and those around him.

In Camus's *The Plague*, whilst ostensibly the story of a vicious epidemic, in reality it is an allegory based on the author's experience of living in France during the German occupation and his being part of the French Resistance. The rats that bring the pestilence to the seaport of Oran are a manifestation of evil that reveal the corruption and inequality of life in the town, the resistance to the plague requiring moral courage to face up to unspeakable crimes that go unchallenged and the need to do and say the right thing in the face of complacency, inertia and social injustice. It is fundamentally a novel about the problem of evil and the existential dilemma of whether we are prepared to do anything about it. After ten years of deliberate austerity that has undermined the resilience of our health-and-social care, and public-health systems, and exacerbated the gross inequality in the country, *The Plague* speaks as loudly to the UK today as it did to its post-World War II audience when it was published in 1947.

Acknowledgements

I wish to place on record my gratitude to all those who have supported me since February 2020 as I have sought to practice public health during the COVID emergency and speak truth to incompetence. This book has been written in close collaboration with my wife, Maggi Morris, former Director of Public Health for Preston and Central Lancashire and interim consultant to the City of Stoke during the pandemic in 2020; her contribution is to be found in many of the pages; most especially the chapter on the cruise liner, the Diamond Princess.

My cousin John Ashton (the other one) has been a constant source of stimulus and challenge; he has influenced my thinking and especially the framing of the responsibility for the UK COVID-19 disaster and what should happen next.

Others who have played in constantly include Ken Spencer, Hugh Lamont, Mick Ord, Dominic Harrison, Julie Hotchkiss, Matt Ashton (who now carries the flame for William Henry Duncan in Liverpool), Gabriel Scally, and other members of the public-health family who had not been intimidated and were prepared to put their heads above the parapets. Lyn Matthews made sure that the voices of the forgotten were remembered. My dear friend Bill Jones was with us in spirit and his wife Jude Yates in person. The Rector of Liverpool, Crispin Pailing of the Parish Church of St Nicholas, Lord David Alton, Lord Nigel Crisp, and Prof. Roger Kirby, President of the Royal Society of Medicine, were important sources of advice and support.

Shelly and Michael Rubinstein, Audrey White, Ken Loach and Michael Sandys gave me invaluable guidance and were of immense moral support when I came under attack, especially after the Panorama expose of government incompetence on BBC TV on 27 April.

Cathy Newman, Alex Crawford and their colleagues at Sky Television; Felicity Lawrence, David Conn and their colleagues at the *Guardian*; Stephen Colegrave, Peter Jukes and Hardeep Matharu at the *Byline Times*; Anthony Casey and Yannis Mendez at Double Down News; Kamran Abbasi at the *Journal of the Royal Society of Medicine*; Fiona Godlee at the *British Medical Journal*; Frea Lockley and Emily Apple at 'The Canary', among other members of the mainstream and new digital media gave me a platform when I was being censored by others. (Whatever you do don't mention BBC Question Time on March 12, I'm still waiting for an apology.)

I am especially grateful to Crown Prince Salman, his colleagues in the Bahrain government and the COVID-19 Task Force led clinically by Lt-Colonel Dr Manaf Al-Quatani for the opportunity to be part of something special.

Many others came forward at personal risk and despite arcane political squabbles to provide me with opportunities to engage with thousands on Zoom and other forms of webinar. I am especially indebted to my close-to 40,000 Twitter followers for their love and support. Some names are held back for fear of recrimination; for others to whom I owe a debt of honour I apologise for your omission.

My families, as always, accepted and supported my diversion during the emergency to this important task.

My publisher, Martin Rynja had faith. I hope he feels it was worth it.

Glossary

Bacteria:
a type of biological cell that may be dangerous when they cause infection

Commensal:
co-existence of organisms in their human or animal host

Endemic:
a disease or condition to be regularly found among a population

Epidemic:
the widespread occurrence of an infectious disease among a population

Epidemiology:
the study of the incidence, distribution and control of the determinants of health and disease

Haemorrhagic fever:
a group of serious illnesses transmitted by families of viruses that include Ebola, Marburg, Lassa and Yellow Fever

Pandemic:
the worldwide spread of a new disease

PHEIC:
Public Health Emergency of International Concern

Prion:
a misfolded protein with the ability to transmit the misfolded shape onto normal variants of the same protein causing transmissible disease

R0:
a measure of the infectivity of an agent. If the R0 is greater than 1.0 each existing infection will cause another one and an epidemic will ensue

Virus:
a sub-microscopic infectious agent that replicates only inside the living cells of an organism

Zoonoses:
diseases that can be spread from animals to humans

Select Bibliography

Ashton, John and Seymour, Howard. *The New Public Health*. Open University Press, 1989.

Ashton, John. *Byline Times* columns, March-July 2020.

Ashton, John. 'COVID-19- One Minute to Midnight'. *BMJ*, March 25th, 2020.

Ashton, John. *Daily Telegraph* February-July 2020.

Ashton, John. Digital newscasts Double Down News, March-July 2020.

Ashton, John. *Journal of the Royal Society of Medicine*, Podium. March-August, 2020.

Ashton, John. *Practising Public Health: An Eyewitness Account*. Oxford University Press, 2019.

Barry, John M. *The Great Influenza. The Epic Story of the Deadliest Plague in History*. Penguin Books, 2004.

Cabinet Office. *Pandemic Influenza LRF Guidance*, July 2013. 'Preparing for Pandemic Influenza, Guidance for Local Planners.'

Camus, Albert. *The Plague*. Penguin, 2013.

Defoe, Daniel. *A Journal of the Plague Year* (1722). Dover Publications, 2003.

Dubois, Rene. *Mirage of Health: Utopias, Progress and Biological Change*. Rutgers University Press, 1987.

Engels, Friedrich. *The Condition of the Working Class in England*, 1845.

Fischetti, Mark. 'Inner workings of the pathogen that has infected the world'. *Scientific American*, July 2020, p28-33.

Hein, Piet. *Grooks*. Hodder and Stoughton, 1969.

Huang, Chaplin et al. 'Clinical features of patients infected with 2019 novel coronavirus in Wuhan, China'. *The Lancet* online, January 24 2020.

Leung, Nancy, et al. 'Respiratory virus shedding in exhaled breath and efficacy of face masks'. *Nature Medicine*, 3 April 2020 26. pp676-680.

McKeown, Thomas. *The Role of Medicine: Dream, Mirage or Nemesis.* Nuffield Provincial Hospitals Trust, 1976.

Owen, David. *The Hubris Syndrome: Bush, Blair and the Intoxication of Power.* Methuen, 2012.

Pickles, W. *Epidemiology in a Country Practice.* John Wright and Son, 1939.

Piot, Peter. *No Time To Lose: A Life in Pursuit of Deadly Viruses.* W.W. Norton & Company, New York, 2012.

Richard Horton, Richard. *The COVID-19 Catastrophe: What's Gone Wrong And How To Stop It Happening Again.* Polity Press, 2020.

Sheard, Sally and Donaldson, Liam. *The Nation's Doctor: The role of the Chief Medical Officer 1855-1998.* The Nuffield Trust, 2006.

Shilts, Randy. *And The Band Played On, Politics, People and the AIDS Epidemic.* Souvenir Press, London, 2007.

Sinclair, Ian and Read, Rupert. 'A National scandal: A Timeline of the UK Government's Woeful Response to the Coronavirus Crisis'. *Byline Times*, 11 April 2020.

'He is at odds with the leading scientists of the UK'
Stephen Barclay MP BBC Question Time 12 March

'John, you are a reasonably lone voice on the panel, I'm not
passing judgement'
Fiona Bruce, Chair BBC Question Time 12h March

'He isn't part of, and doesn't speak for, nor represent the view of
the public-health community, Nor is he involved in developing
public-health policy'
Greg Fell, Director of Public Health, Sheffield, 12 March

'The Chief Medical Officer and his team have the 100% support
and backing of the Public Health Community. Every DPH I
know thinks he is doing an amazing job in difficult circumstances. Sorry but JRA is just demonstrating he is out of touch
on this'
Greg Fell, Director of Public Health, Sheffield 12 March

'I'm glad John is not leading our response at COBR… I'm glad
John is not involved in the decision-making tree… Because John
is ill-informed and what he is doing is the exact opposite of what
leading medical professions (*sic*) should be doing, which is be
looking and supporting government… which is supporting
decisions that they make which is the right decisions at the right
time for us'.
Dr Clare Gerada Channel 4 News, 14 March 2020

'It pains me to say it, but the UK public health community (with the exception of Professor John Ashton and a few others) have some very serious questions to answer. They clearly backed the herd immunity stance of the CMO and CSO.'
Dr Clive Peedell

'It will be like those American movies, where the mad scientist was right all along'
Dominic Harrison, Director of Public Health
Blackburn with Darwen, March 2020.

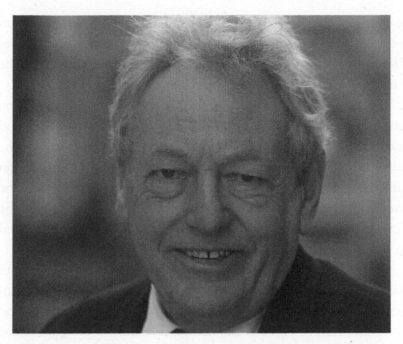

Professor John Ashton is one of Britain's foremost public-health consultants. Born in Liverpool and educated as a medical doctor at the University of Newcastle upon Tyne and the London School of Hygiene and Tropical Medicine, he specialised in psychiatry, general practice and sexual health before training in public health.

In a career extending over 50 years he has been one of the pioneers of what came to be known as The New Public Health. His book of the same name, co-authored with Howard Seymour in 1989, became the standard textbook for a generation of public health students and his recent book *Practising Public Health, an Eyewitness Account* (Oxford University Press, 2019) brings together the experiences from his many highly acclaimed interventions and innovations in the field of public health at local, national and global levels. These include pioneering large-scale health promotion efforts on lifestyle change, reducing teenage pregnancy rates and the first large scale syringe exchange programme for intravenous drug users in the face of the epidemic of HIV/AIDS in the 1980's which led to the global adoption of what came to be known as 'harm reduction'. He was one of the founders of the WHO Healthy Cities Project in 1986 and continues to work as senior consultant to the European Healthy Cities Network over 30 years later.

Professor Ashton's style of practice is renowned for being hands-on as well as 'big picture'. As a Liverpool supporter and spectator at the Hillsborough Football Stadium disaster in 1989 he implemented triage of the dying and injured in the absence of an effective emergency response and was the first to champion the truth about the disaster in the face of malicious efforts to blame the fans and the victims themselves as a number of those in charge tried to cover up their own responsibility.

In 1999, as a member of the British humanitarian delegation to Kosovo at the end of the civil war in the Balkans he intervened personally with US President Bill Clinton in the refugee camps and persuaded him to evacuate almost 200 seriously ill refugees to the US when the international agencies were withdrawing. He was awarded the CBE by Prime Minister Tony Blair for services to the NHS. His intervention on behalf of NHS staff in the fuel protests at Stanlow Oil Refinery that had brought the country to a standstill, resulted in the protesters lifting their blockade.

Since February 2020, at the request of Bahrain's Deputy Prime Minister Crown Prince Salman he has been acting as a critical friend in the Bahraini COVID-19 Task Force which has been praised by the Director General of the WHO for its outstanding performance in dealing with the epidemic.

Throughout his career John has practised Professor Geoffrey Rose's call for public health workers to have 'a clean mind and dirty hands' always bridging the worlds of academia and hands on practice. He is a visiting professor at the Liverpool school of Tropical Medicine, the London School of Hygiene and Tropical Medicine, the University of Liverpool, Liverpool John Moores University and the University of Cumbria among others.

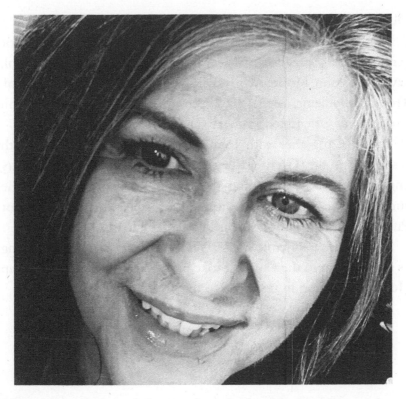

Maggi Morris is one of the new breed of public health consultants who comes from a non-traditional background in the humanities. After studying anthropology at Reading University, she worked in the University of Liverpool School of Architecture for twenty years with a special interest in housing and prisons.

After training in public health in the 1990s she became one of the first non-medical Directors of Public Health, working for eleven years in Preston and Central Lancashire where she was Director of Children's Health and Wellbeing for Lancashire. She was instrumental in bringing the experience of 'Smoke Free California' to the UK and made significant contributions in developing a public health approach to primary care and Asset Based Community Development, as one of the protégés of one of its founders John McKnight who had been a trainer of Barack

Obama as a community organiser in Chicago.

Most recently, Maggi has been providing leadership training for senior health professionals at Manchester Business School, Liverpool John Moores University and the Liverpool School of Tropical Medicine. Maggi has been an adviser to the WHO on Community Orientated Primary Care.

In 2018, together with John Ashton, she led a public health response to the Grenfell Tower tragedy based on community engagement and monitoring the impact of the tragedy on the survivors and bereaved and others affected. She was a Senior Public-Health Advisor at Kensington and Chelsea Council.

During the pandemic of COVID-19 Maggi has been working as a consultant in the City of Stoke public-health team, heading up Health Protection in response to the virus.